Stability

Ball

A Guide for

Fitness

Professionals

Training

from the

American

Council

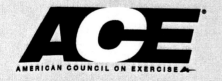

on Exercise

ISBN: 1-58518-723-2
Library of Congress Control Number: 2002111212

Distributed by:
American Council on Exercise
P.O. Box 910449
San Diego, CA 92191-0449
(858) 279-8227
(858) 279-8064 (FAX)
www.ACEfitness.org

Author: Sabra Bonelli
Managing Editor: Daniel Green
Technical Editor: Cedric X. Bryant, Ph.D.
Design & Production: Karen McGuire
Director of Publications: Christine J. Ekeroth
Associate Editor: Lisa Frantz Adlam
Editorial Assistant: Jennifer Schiffer
Index: Bonny McLaughlin
Models: Doug Balzarini, DeeDee Kovacevich, Al Mirnezam, & Beckie Page
Photography: Dennis Dal Covey

Acknowledgments:
Thanks to the entire American Council on Exercise staff for their support and guidance through the process of creating this manual.

NOTICE
The fitness industry is ever-changing. As new research and clinical experience broaden our knowledge, changes in programming and standards are required. The authors and the publisher of this work have checked with sources believed to be reliable in their efforts to provide information that is complete and generally in accord with the standards accepted at the time of publication. However, in view of the possibility of human error or changes in industry standards, neither the authors nor the publisher nor any other party who has been involved in the preparation or publication of this work warrants that the information contained herein is in every respect accurate or complete, and they are not responsible for any errors or omissions or the results obtained from the use of such information. Readers are encouraged to confirm the information contained herein with other sources.

Published by:
Healthy Learning
P.O. Box 1828
Monterey, CA 93942
(888) 229-5745
(831) 372-6075 (Fax)
www.healthylearning.com

Christine Cunningham is the owner of performENHANCE sport and adventure athlete training in Chicago. She is an ACE-certified Personal Trainer, an NSCA-certified C.S.C.S., and NATA-certified athletic trainer. Cunningham is a member of the Life Fitness Academy and ACE Faculty Advisory Board. She is a frequent industry lecturer and writer and is currently a Ph.D. candidate in motor control and learning at the University of Illinois at Chicago.

Mike Morris, B.A., R.T.S., C.P.F.T., holds a bachelor of arts degree from Nicholls State University in Louisiana and is a Master Level Resistance Specialist of Resistance University, Oklahoma City, Okla. He is an NASM-certified personal trainer and a continuing education provider for ACE, NASM, ACSM, NDEITA, NCSF, AEA, and AFAA. Morris is an international presenter with many organizations, as well as a 4-star presenter with IDEA. Mike and his wife, Stephanie, are founders of the Resist-A-Ball®, program and creators of the Resist-A-Ball® C.O.R.E. Instructor Certification Program.

Carol Murphy is the owner and fitness director of Fitlife in Rochester, New York. She is a member of the ACE Academy as a Continuing Education Specialist, and is a Master Trainer for Resist-A-Ball® and Reebok University. Her certifications include ACSM, ACE, and AFAA. Murphy is an international presenter and co-star of two stability ball videos.

Joan Wenson is an ACE-certified Personal Trainer and co-founder of Peloton Fitness, a professional organization aimed at fostering the growth and longevity of indoor cycling through programming within health clubs worldwide. Wenson is also the director of education at LeMond Academy, where she designs group exercise programs and has partnered with Greg LeMond on four videos for cycling enthusiasts. She currently teaches various group exercise classes — including stability ball training — that draw on her careers in ballet and performance aerobics.

CONTENTS

INTRODUCTION

The American Council on Exercise (ACE) is pleased to introduce *Stability Ball Training,* a guide for fitness professionals. The stability ball has emerged in recent years as one of the fitness industry's most versatile and widely used pieces of equipment. The intent of this book is to educate and give guidance to personal trainers that wish to train clients using the stability ball in a one-on-one setting, as well as group fitness instructors teaching stability ball classes or incorporating balls into other types of classes. As with all areas of fitness, education is a continual process. ACE recognizes this is a broad subject requiring serious study and we encourage you to use the References and Suggested Reading to further your knowledge.

Introduction to Stability Ball Training

Known by many names, from Swiss Ball to Gymnastic Ball to Physioball, the "stability ball" is arguably the most versatile and useful piece of exercise equipment to enter the fitness arena in more than a decade. The stability ball is a large, inflated vinyl rubber ball that comes in a variety of sizes, colors, and even shapes. Its most common use is, not surprisingly, in the area of balance training, with advocates continually promoting core musculature stabilization. In addition, the stability ball is a valuable exercise tool that offers cardiovascular, muscle strength, muscle endurance, and flexibility training for the entire body. Most importantly, this is an exercise prop that is both challenging and fun, offering options to exercisers of virtually all skill and ability levels.

History and Growth

Contrary to what many fitness professionals might think, the stability ball is not a new invention. In fact, use of the ball began in the physical therapy arena more than 90 years ago. The stability ball was first used by Dr. Susanne Klein-Vogelbach in Switzerland in 1909, where it came to be known as the Swiss Ball. Dr. Klein-Vogelbach introduced the Swiss Ball in her physical therapy work with children with cerebral palsy, helping them to maintain reflex response as well as improve their balance. Recognizing the value of the ball, the physical therapy community used it in the treatment of neurological and orthopedic disorders as well as spinal injuries. The ball made its appearance in the United States in the late 1970s and early 1980s, where it continued to be used as an exercise, balance, and therapy aid in the medical rehab arena, primarily by physical therapists. It is only in the past decade that the stability ball made the transition to the fitness industry.

In 1992 Mike and Stephanie Morris developed a total-body fitness-training program around the ball and are credited by many as having led the way for use of the stability ball in both the group exercise and personal training fields. Their Resist-A-Ball® program introduced this unique piece of exercise equipment, along with an extensive educational program, to the mainstream health and fitness market. Since then the stability ball has become a staple in fitness facilities across the country and, indeed, around the world. A variety of different resources, including books, videos, and fitness professional training programs and seminars, have been developed. Since that time, many other fitness professionals have been instrumental in bringing stability ball exercise into the traditional fitness and performance training arenas.

The past five years have shown a dramatic rise in stability ball usage both in facilities and privately in home gyms and even offices. This may be attributed to an increasing body of research recognizing the effectiveness of stability ball training as well as media coverage increasing the public's awareness of this fitness modality. A survey of fitness programming trends in 2000 by *IDEA Health and Fitness Source* revealed that 60% of fitness facilities offer stability ball–based group exercise classes, compared to the 16% reported in 1996 (IDEA, 2001). Further, when survey respondents were asked how often stability balls are used in group exercise classes, they responded with a staggering 75%. This reveals that stability balls are frequently used during portions of other group exercise classes in addition to "stability ball classes" (IDEA, 2001). Use of the stability ball in personal training has experienced similar growth as industry trends move toward functional, core, and balance training.

Those in the fitness-savvy baby-boomer generation, who fully experienced the era of bodybuilding and aerobic dance, recognize the need for maintaining quality of life. They have watched their parents and grandparents struggle with everyday functional movements and are seeking ways to avoid a similar fate as they head into their golden years. The fitness industry has responded with a push toward exercising for functional fitness, which includes training for balance, coordination, and flexibility. Further, with the myriad of benefits stability ball training offers for all segments of the population, it is advisable that fitness professionals become familiar and comfortable with the use of this versatile training tool.

Benefits

The stability ball is perhaps the most versatile piece of equipment currently available, as it utilizes the neuromuscular system in a way that most other exercise equipment does not, requiring the integrated involvement of strength, flexibility, and balance. Ball exercises are designed primarily to enhance the exerciser's ability to move the body without restrictions and to perform functional movements necessary to meet the needs and challenges of daily life. Regular use of the stability ball can give users an improved quality of life as they develop the strength, flexibility, and balance to work and play without movement limitations.

One of the greatest benefits of stability ball usage is improved balance. The ball challenges the individual to develop the ability to continually balance and focuses effort on the core stabilizer muscles (the abdominals, low back, and hips/pelvis), regardless of the movement being performed. To train on the ball requires balance and motor control, both of which will improve through regular use of the ball. Exercises can be designed to work solely on balance, while other exercises can work on strengthening and/or stretching practically any muscle group in the body. The best feature of the ball is that while strength or flexibility work is being performed, balance work is taking place simultaneously. No muscle or muscle group can be targeted in isolation to the exclusion of the stabilizing muscles that balance the body. This time-efficient training feature makes stability ball exercises challenging and beneficial to users of all skill and ability levels.

Probably the most publicized and well-known benefit of stability ball training is that the balls allow exercisers to train and develop strength and tone of the trunk musculature, particularly the abdominals. A recent study at San Diego State University used electromyography (EMG) equipment to examine muscle activity in 13 common abdominal exercises. Crunches on the stability ball ranked third overall in abdominal muscle activity. However, there was less activity in the hip flexor muscles during ball crunches than the bicycle maneuver and the Captain's

Chair exercise, which were ranked number one and two in the study, respectively. As hip flexion during abdominal work indicates that the exercise does not isolate the abdominals preferentially, researchers concluded that crunches on the stability ball arguably are the most effective abdominal exercise overall (American Council on Exercise, 2001). It is no wonder then that stability balls are a top pick for home exercise equipment, due to their low cost, high level of effectiveness, and versatility.

Another benefit of the ball is its demand for any movement to be performed with correct posture. Proper posture with neutral spinal alignment is a necessity as the stabilizer muscles of the core work to balance the body on the ball. Regular use of the stability ball improves spinal stability as the core stabilizer muscles become stronger at adapting to an unstable base of support. Chronically bad posture is one of the main causes of muscle imbalance that leads to low-back pain, which is statistically likely to be experienced by more than three-quarters of the adult population at some point in their lives (Darragh, 1999). Improved posture through stability ball training can be a very effective way of preventing or relieving low-back pain.

Due to the constant posture and balance training required to perform movements, stability ball training is different from, and in many ways superior to, traditional strength-training methods. To fully appreciate the value of stability ball training, one must understand that the human body functions as a coordinated unit, with muscles contracting in proper sequence (i.e., some contracting to help balance the body, others contracting to stabilize critical areas of the body such as the spine, and still others contracting in response to external stimuli such as a sudden change in body position or a loss of balance). Using the unstable surface of the ball, the body has to work as one coordinated unit, moving with proper body mechanics at all times to maintain correct form and posture. If movements are jerky or uncoordinated, the goals of functional strengthening are limited, posture breaks down, balance is challenged, and the user may even lose equilibrium and fall. The advantage to stability ball training is that the balance challenge can be easily modified to appropriate levels of progression by varying the body position or ball size or firmness.

One of the greatest benefits of regular stability ball training is its effect on everyday life, yielding improved quality of life with better functioning, decreased risk of injury, and improved posture and balance. Because ball training involves balance, posture, and moving as a coordinated unit, it is ultimately, as previously mentioned, functional fitness training. Much of traditional fitness training, while certainly effective at improving cardiorespiratory function, muscle strength, and flexibility, involves movement in a stable environment. Stability balls challenge the body to react and learn to move efficiently in an unstable environment. As so much of real-life motion involves adapting to changing conditions, such as when playing soccer, gardening, or carrying groceries upstairs, ball work is exceptional for improving functional abilities.

From a programming and instruction perspective, stability ball training is of great value to both personal trainers and group fitness instructors. First and foremost is the endless variety of exercises available on the ball. There are innumerable ways to functionally strengthen virtually every muscle group in the body. In addition, stability ball training can be very time-efficient. For example, it is possible to sufficiently overload muscles in less time than with non-ball exercises because core training and balance work occur as other muscle groups are trained. This allows for the targeting of more muscle groups when time is limited. Additionally, the stability ball is useful for accommodating multiple ability levels in one class. Any exercise on the ball can be easily and quickly adapted to the individual needs of each participant. One further benefit of ball training is that the curved surface of the ball allows for positions and movement patterns that simply are not possible on the floor. This enables exercisers to move through all three planes of motion for a more functional challenge than is offered by traditional exercises.

From the exerciser's perspective, the ball is light-weight, fun, and low-tech. The stability ball is large and colorful and has a comforting shape, which promotes a sense of play that makes exercise fun and interesting. Laughter is often one of the first responses from novice stability ball users, before they realize how challenging exercise on the ball can be. The endless variety of exercises possible on the ball also helps counteract boredom. Many fitness enthusiasts find themselves intimidated by complex exercises and awkward equipment. The ball is extremely user-friendly, as it supports and eases the body into proper posture and exercise positions. It is also simple to vary the resistive and/or balance challenge within each exercise by simply changing body position on the ball.

Stability balls also are extremely durable and adaptable for use with just about any population. Because stability balls have been shown to have positive results with people with a wide variety of diagnosed medical conditions, there are very few, if any, "special populations" for which the ball is inappropriate. Use of the ball for strength or stretch work can be safe and effective for just about any condition, provided the exercises are chosen well. It is critical that you are familiar with the variety of common conditions and injuries and know what types of movements are most suitable to each population. Considerations and contraindications are

Table 1.1

HEIGHT	BALL SIZE
Under 4'6" (137 cm)	30 cm (12 inches)
4'6" to 5'0" (137 to 152 cm)	45 cm (18 inches)
5'1" to 5'7" (155 to 170 cm)	55 cm (22 inches)
5'8" to 6'2" (173 to 188 cm)	65 cm (26 inches)
Over 6'2" (188 cm)	75 cm (30 inches)

presented for specific groups and conditions in Chapter Five.

Choosing the Right Stability Ball

The stability ball should be selected for use according to each individual's height. Ball size is the diameter of the ball as measured from the floor up to peak height (measured in centimeters). Use Table 1.1 as a guide for determining the proper ball size to use for strength and flexibility work.

Heavier people and those with especially long limbs might benefit from the next larger size, regardless of these height guidelines. It should be noted that there is also an 85 cm (34 inch) stability ball available for heavier or long-legged exercisers who find the 75 cm ball uncomfortable.

In all cases it is your responsibility to guide exercisers to choose the correct size and firmness ball for their individual skill levels. Extremely firm balls provide less resistance to movement and roll more easily and quickly. These balls make exercises more challenging and are appropriate for more advanced exercisers who have experience with balance training. A less firm ball that is somewhat deflated creates a wider base of support for the exerciser because more of the surface of the ball is in contact with the ground. These less-inflated balls make exercises easier and are appropriate for beginning exercisers, deconditioned individuals, older adults, and persons who are particularly challenged with balance training. Softer balls also are more comfortable for large, heavier people who need to balance more body weight during ball exercise.

Inflation Information

With the purchase of the stability ball comes one or more ball plugs, and an inflation adapter for use with a bicycle pump or an electric air pump, such as those for inflating basketballs, or for use with the air compressor at gas stations. Inflate balls according to size. Once balls are inflated to complete fullness, air can be released to adjust the firmness of the ball, depending on the needs of the exerciser. Some balls also come with a plug remover, or one can be purchased separately.

The selection of stability balls available for group fitness classes should include balls with varying degrees of firmness, especially as most facilities do not provide the entire range of ball sizes listed above. Help participants select a ball inflated to the point that best suits their individual skill and ability levels, in addition to meeting the needs of their limb length. Ultimately, each person needs a stability ball that allows them to sit with their knees aligned with their hips so the knees form a 90-degree angle when the feet are flat on the floor with the ankles under the knees.

It should be noted that regular use of the stability ball stretches the vinyl. Periodically check ball size and firmness and add air to ensure proper inflation.

Storage and Cleaning

The shape and size of stability balls make storage a challenge in most health club environments, as deflating and re-inflating the balls for each use is too time consuming and inconvenient. Various types of storage racks are available for purchase. Additionally, there are balls made with legs (also called udders), which are three-inch-long thumb-sized protrusions of inflated vinyl in one area of the ball (usually near the plug). With legs, stability balls can be stacked up to three balls high. Another option is to purchase a net that can contain the balls in one area of the exercise room.

Washing the stability balls in water or mild soapy water is the ideal way to clean the vinyl surface. Do not use chemical cleaners that are harsh or abrasive, as they will damage the covering. Balls should be washed regularly for comfort and sanitary reasons, since the surface can get dirty from consistent contact with the floor. To help preserve the life of the balls, keep the exercise room floor clean and free of sharp objects. Replace any balls that cannot hold air or on which the vinyl has been damaged from sharp objects.

Traditional stability balls are very durable and suitable for most environments. "Burst resistant" balls are made with a material that will deflate very slowly when punctured rather than bursting like a balloon (depending on the size of the puncture). Some facilities prefer these balls to avoid any problems should a ball be punctured.

Environment and Space Requirements

Facility standards and guidelines from the American College of Sports Medicine state that participants in any group exercise class should be spaced six feet apart (American College of Sports Medicine, 1997, a). The ideal situation for stability ball usage is for each exerciser to have an entire body's length of space clear in all directions around the ball. Depending on the total room or class size, this can be very challenging—and in some cases, impossible. To accommodate a stability ball class in which participants need to be closer to one another than is optimal, make sure all participants transition simultaneously when rolling back, forward, or to the side for an exercise.

There is no one preferred floor surface recommended for stability ball training. The ball is made of material that works well on every surface from wood floors to carpet. When working on a hard surface, keep in mind the need for support and cushion for the parts of the body in contact with the floor, such as the knees, thighs, and forearms, depending on the exercise selected. Advise participants to keep an exercise mat nearby for these situations. Yoga "sticky" mats work well to keep participants from sliding in certain positions, such as side-lying or prone over the ball during trunk extension.

The room environment for stability ball training should be no different than normally provided for strength or flexibility training. Moderately warmer temperatures [68°F to 72°F (20°C to 22°C)] are appropriate for workouts emphasizing only flexibility or for yoga on the ball. Cooler temperatures [60°F to 67°F (16°C to 19°C)] are suitable for strength training or workouts incorporating both strength and flexibility.

Attire

Guidelines for proper attire for stability ball exercises promote the safest and most comfortable use possible. It should be noted that bare skin contacting the ball surface interferes with smooth movement. Exposed skin can stick uncomfortably to the vinyl covering, while perspiring skin may be slippery. Both situations hinder continuous and flowing movement. For this reason, wearing very short shorts (such as running shorts) and using the ball with uncovered skin, such as in a bra-top

without a T-shirt, is not recommended. Depending on the type of moves being performed, a small towel can be draped on the ball to reduce contact between skin and vinyl. Preferable apparel selections include long leggings, longer shorts, cotton shirts, and tight-fitting clothing that is moisture-wicking or made of materials such as Lycra, spandex, or Supplex. Large, loose-fitting clothing is discouraged, as it can get in the way of smooth movements, be slippery against the ball, and hinder your ability to view exercisers' body alignment during exercises.

Footwear is an important part of stability ball work. Athletic shoes are required for proper ball use. Socks with shoes off should be discouraged at all times, as socks tend to be slippery against the floor and ball and can lead to a fall or injury. The type of athletic shoe is not critical. It simply needs to be a close-toed exercise shoe designed to support and protect the foot during exercise. Shoes also provide stability for the feet, allowing for strong and safe contact with the floor during the workout. Bare feet can also provide appropriate points of contact with the floor during stability ball exercises and are most suitable for workouts focusing on yoga or flexibility training.

Exercise Science

CHAPTER TWO

To safely and effectively incorporate stability balls into your programming, you must have a good understanding of certain basic concepts and exercise principles as they apply to ball training and be familiar with the importance of balance and why regular balance training is crucial to every person's fitness routine. It is also important you understand the design and function of the core musculature and have a good working knowledge of proper biomechanics for ball training along with the effects of gravity and body positioning for designing stability ball exercises. The principles of appropriate overload and proper progression are key when teaching stability ball exercise. Exercisers should be able to hold a base position with proper form and alignment before an additional challenge is provided through balance work or external resistance. This base of knowledge will provide you with all the tools necessary to design and cue stability ball exercises correctly so workouts are challenging and productive with minimal risk of injury.

Core Strength and Stability

In virtually every movement performed, the core musculature stabilizes the rest of the body. The core, or trunk, muscles, consisting of the abdominals and back, are the link between the upper and lower halves of the body. All actions should involve the core as the foundation for movements, as it is these muscles that are the center of power for the body and the origin of movement. Movements that do not recruit the core muscles for power are inefficient, awkward, and sometimes dangerous. Because the muscles supporting the spine have been trained to activate appropriately just prior to movement, a strong core allows one to move the body with varying loads while the spine is stabilized. Deconditioned people and many low-back pain sufferers have trouble stabilizing themselves for movement because of their inability to properly activate the muscles that support the spine. It should be noted that there is an inner unit of core muscles that are local stabilizers (multifidus, diaphragm, pelvic floor, quadratus lumborum, etc.), but it is the large outer core trunk muscles (the global movers)

that will be reviewed and referenced in this publication.

It is important to have a clear understanding of what core stability is all about. The word core means "the central or inner part, the essence or most important part of a matter," while stability is "the capacity of an object to return to equilibrium or to its original position after being displaced" (Creager & Creswell, 2000). Core stability, then, is the ability to stay balanced while shifting weight or moving the body from its center of gravity. The central nervous system is the starting point for balanced movement, which begins with the intrinsic or core stabilizing muscles. These are the muscles responsible for posture, joint stability, and mobility. There are numerous muscles that work in the core to stabilize the spine and allow effective movement. The most significant are these intrinsic muscles: the rectus abdominis, the internal and external obliques, the transverse abdominis, and the erector spinae. The muscles of the chest and pelvis are also active in core movement, but the true trunk stabilizers are the abdominals and back (Figure 2.1).

The most superficial abdominal muscle is the rectus abdominis, also known as the "six pack" because of the naturally occurring segments of muscle connected by flat tendons that make up the rectus muscle. This muscle acts to both flex and rotate the lumbar spine,

Figure 2.1

Muscles of the abdominal wall

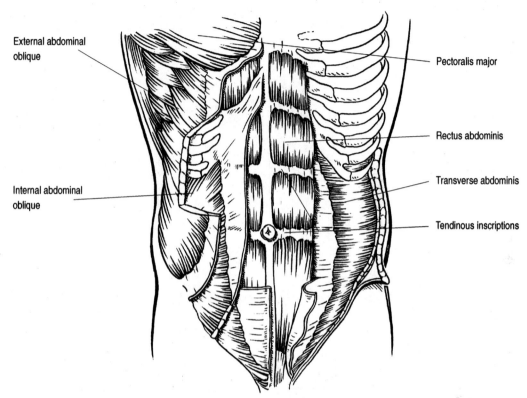

External abdominal oblique

Internal abdominal oblique

Pectoralis major

Rectus abdominis

Transverse abdominis

Tendinous inscriptions

stabilize the pelvis during walking, and increase intra-abdominal pressure.

The innermost muscle of the abdominal region is the transverse abdominis, which contains the deepest fibers of the abdominal wall. This muscle works to compress the abdominal cavity, which is important for increased trunk stability and proper posture maintenance.

The fibers of the internal and external obliques run diagonally across the torso, perpendicular to one another, from the outer edges of the ribs toward the midline of the body. The role of these muscles, which make up the sides of the abdominal area, is twofold. When the obliques on both sides of the body contract simultaneously, these muscles aid the rectus abdominis muscle in flexing the spine and compressing the abdomen. When the internal obliques on one side of the body and the external obliques on the opposite side of the body are contracted, these muscles work with the back to perform trunk rotation or to laterally flex the spine.

The back muscles collectively make up the erector spinae group, which consists of three muscle columns that run the length of the spine from the lower back: the longissimus, the iliocostalis, and the spinalis. The erector spinae muscles are the principle movers of the back and function to perform back extension and lateral flexion of the vertebral column to maintain posture. Strong postural muscles and proper posture are key factors in relieving and preventing low-back pain (YMCA of the USA, 2001). Research indicates that 80% of the North American population will experience back pain at some point in their lives; therefore, proper conditioning of the erector spinae muscles is critical (IDEA, 1999).

There is a variety of core-strengthening movements available to exercisers. The core musculature creates and shifts power to the extremities of the upper- and lower-body, while also stabilizing the lumbar spine and pelvis. With such a wide scope of responsibilities, core muscles require proper training that includes many different exercises that address the various actions of each of the core muscles. The stability ball is the most versatile tool for providing core strengthening options that address the many different tasks the core muscles are called upon to perform in daily activities. See page 59 for a detailed presentation of core-strengthening exercises.

Balance

Balance is an extremely important, but often overlooked, component in a well-designed exercise program. It is a basic movement skill required to maintain equilibrium and keep the body upright and able to move. Ultimately, balance is a function of the nervous system, whereby the senses, especially the eyes, ears, and internal proprioception skills (awareness of our body in space), signal the nervous system about our body position and the need to make changes if balance is compromised. Noted physical therapist Deborah Ellison explains in an article written for the Web by Karen Asp that every move the human body makes requires balance. She defines balance as "simply keeping your center of gravity within your base of support. If you know where your center is, that is your body unconsciously knowing where, then you're more grounded physically and mentally."

Balance training gives exercisers the chance to practice maintaining equilibrium and thereby avoid injury. When an external stimulus signals the nervous system that balance is compromised, such as when you step on something slippery and lose your footing while walking, a quick reaction time is needed for the body to adjust, regain balance, and avoid falling. Most likely, someone who has trained to improve balance will have a

Table 2.1 — Internal and External Factors Affecting Balance

INTERNAL FACTORS: Can be broken down into two categories: physiological and psychological.

Physiological:
- physical fitness (endurance, strength, flexibility, agility, coordination)
- kinesthetic awareness
- visual perception
- vestibular system
- existing motor skills/reflexes
- posture
- stance
- improper warm-up/excessive training

Psychological:
- self-confidence
- courage
- adaptability
- mental control
- commitment
- anxiety
- fear
- expectations
- peer pressure

EXTERNAL FACTORS:
- improperly fitted equipment (shoes or other)
- gravity
- friction
- speed
- obstacles
- terrain irregularities
- weather conditions

Source: Nottingham (1999). Reprinted with permission from IDEA Health and Fitness Association, the leading international membership association in the health and fitness industry.

quicker reaction time, and will be more likely to regain balance with proper form and alignment, than someone who has not practiced maintaining their body position in an unstable environment. Outdoor fitness training expert Suzanne Nottingham writes, "Through balance conditioning, clients learn how to automatically respond to a sense of imbalance. This in turn allows them to learn new movement skills and move more efficiently during all activities" (Nottingham, 1999). Table 2.1 lists of a variety of internal and external factors that influence balance.

Stability ball training addresses almost all of the internal and external factors listed in Table 2.1 to train the body for improved balance. For example, one of the internal physiological factors is physical fitness. Regular use of the stability ball improves core muscle strength, muscle endurance, and flexi-bility, which improve overall physical fitness and aid the body's ability to balance. Posture is another internal physiological factor the ball addresses. Work on the ball is difficult if not impossible to perform correctly unless the spine is neutral. Although some exercises (suspended prone positions that load spinal flexion, push-ups, or roll-out positions) are safer taught with a slight posterior pelvic tilt for beginners who may fatigue and easily release into an excessively curved lumbar position, neutral spine is crucial during stability ball exercises. Also, core work on the ball trains the small stabilizer muscles that affect posture. Improved posture helps the body balance more easily.

Two common concerns related to stability ball training are fear and lack of self-confidence. Many people, especially older adults and larger-sized individuals, have a great fear of falling and little confidence in their ability to prevent themselves from falling (American Council on Exercise, 1998). Work on the stability ball, performed correctly and progressed appropriately, teaches exercisers that they can challenge themselves in an unstable environment confidently and without fear. This translates to improved balance and less hesitancy during real-life movements that require balance adjustments.

External factors such as gravity and movement speed also are involved in ball training. See page 17 for a discussion of gravity's role in stability ball training. Movement speed is used to alter the difficulty level of an exercise or target a specific activity more effectively. Movements that occur faster on the ball require great coordination and agility. At the same time, they also can involve momentum if not performed correctly, rendering the exercise less effective. For example, a common mistake seen with trunk curls involves bouncing off the ball into flexion, as opposed to using control to make a deliberate movement. Progress clients appropriately from first holding a position with good form, alignment, and balance before adding movement. Agility and coordination improvements cannot take place without good balance.

There are two kinds of balance that can be worked on: static and dynamic. Static balance involves stillness, which is the ability to hold the body in place. An example of static balance is standing on one leg. The ball can be used to train static balance, which gets better with improved posture, muscle strength, and flexibility. Dynamic balance requires coordination to balance while the body is moving, such as when walking. All people use both static and dynamic balance throughout their daily lives. Although we think more often of balance as static, it is dynamic balance that is more often involved in falls and injuries and is what most people need to improve. The stability ball is ultimately designed to train for dynamic balance and thereby improve functional fitness for activities of daily living, as well as to train athletes to improve performance with better coordination, agility, strength, endurance, and flexibility.

One of the simplest ways to train for dynamic balance is to have clients adjust their base of support when performing an exercise on the ball. For example, performing abdominal crunches on the ball with the feet on the floor hip-distance apart is standard. To increase the challenge, have them bring their feet closer together or even lift one foot from the floor, making a smaller base of support and requiring greater balance work from the core musculature. A different way of working dynamic balance on the stability ball is to move the ball during an exercise. For example, the latissimus dorsi can be worked by rolling the ball away from the core. In this exercise,

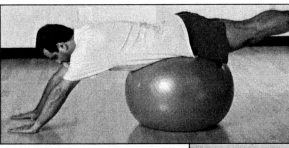

Figure 2.2
a. Rolling lat pull start position, arms extended

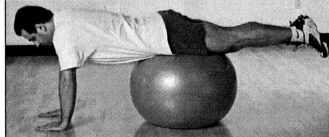

b. Ending position, wrists under shoulders

an exerciser begins lying prone over the ball with the ball under the hips. The legs are lifted off the ground and the arms extended overhead, the palms resting on the floor shoulder-width apart. The lat work occurs as the exerciser pulls the body forward until the shoulders are in line with the palms. The ball rolls from under the hips to under the thighs, knees, or shins, depending on limb length. Here dynamic balance is required to keep the body centered while both the body and the ball are moving (Figure 2.2).

Biomechanics

One of the greatest results that can come from stability ball use is improved posture, or body alignment. Biomechanically correct posture involves relaxed knees, a neutral pelvis, lifted chest, retracted shoulders, and a neutral head. Work on the ball requires moving (or being still) while in neutral spinal alignment. Many people have poor posture due to sedentary lifestyles that have deconditioned their postural muscles so that the trunk muscles are not strong enough to support the body in the most efficient way. Essentially, the neuro-muscular system has "unlearned" how to easily and properly maintain posture. This weak core creates a situation where chances of injury are increased. The stability ball works to correct postural alignment by requiring balance. To balance on the ball, the body's own support mechanisms must be used as there is no external support available for assistance. When balance is challenged, the body's automatic response is to activate the equilibrium mechanism, which coordinates postural muscles so balance is maintained with the least amount of effort. With no external support, the easiest position that provides balance is neutral spinal alignment and proper posture. Each movement on the ball requires body awareness and encourages self-reliance and confidence in the body's ability to balance itself. The more often one works out on the ball, the better the body's motor control becomes. The result is a heightened awareness of the central nervous system that helps to maintain neutral spinal alignment and reduce likelihood of injury.

The ability to teach neutral spinal alignment is important in working with the stability ball. To better understand neutral spinal alignment, low-back movements must be considered in relationship to the pelvis. A pelvic tilt can occur in an anterior, posterior, or lateral direction. Neutral is different for everyone, but it lies somewhere between anterior and posterior without movement in the lateral direction and places minimal stress on the spine. From neck to tailbone, a neutral spine involves a slight inward curve, or extension, at the neck, a slight outward curve, or flexion, in the thoracic spine (chest and rib area), and a slight inward curve, or lordosis, in the lumbar spine (Darragh, 1999). Holding the neutral spinal position requires strong core muscles that can function in a coordinated manner. The neutral spine position is challenged anytime the pelvis is tilted too far in one direction or

when any one of the core muscles is either too strong or too weak in relationship to the others, which results in a misinterpretation of nervous system signals (Figure 2.3). Regularly maintaining the spine outside of one's neutral alignment increases chances of back pain and problems such as a degenerative disk, pinched nerves, and bulging disks (Darragh, 1999). It is crucial then that body alignment be correct during exercise, which will lead to proper body alignment in everyday activities.

The seated position on the ball provides an excellent opportunity to teach neutral spinal alignment and posterior, anterior, and lateral tilt. As was discussed in Chapter One, clients should be seated on a ball inflated enough to allow for 90-degree angles at both the hips and knees. Once seated on the appropriately sized ball, have them perform small anterior and posterior pelvic tilts to get used to the feeling of moving on the ball. Ask them to roll the ball slightly forward by tilting the pelvis posteriorly, or to roll the ball slightly backward by tilting the pelvis anteriorly. These pelvic tilts should be followed by smaller-to-larger hip circles, as clients continue to experience moving and balancing on the ball. These rolling actions help clients visually and physically connect to the movement pattern. Bouncing on the ball from the seated position may also give a feel for balancing during ball exercise. Neutral spinal alignment occurs when clients can balance and rest in the seated

Figure 2.3
Pelvic tilt can be anterior, posterior, or lateral. The bucket of water serves as a visual aid to better illustrate the direction of the pelvic tilt.

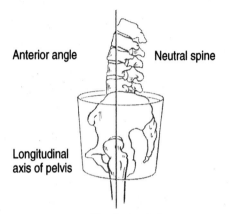

Neutral pelvis
Neutral lumbar spine with neutral pelvis.

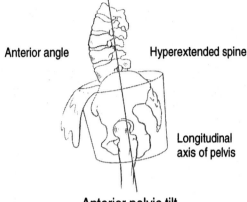

Anterior pelvic tilt
Lumbar hyperextension with anterior pelvic tilt.

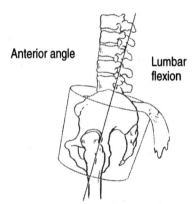

Posterior pelvic tilt
Slight lumbar flexion with posterior pelvic tilt.

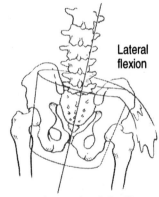

Lateral pelvic tilt
Lateral lumbar flexion with lateral pelvic tilt.

position on the ball with the spine elongated with natural curvatures in the neck, thoracic, and lumbar regions. Although many may have difficulty finding the neutral working position challenging at first, reassure them that finding and moving in neutral becomes easier, and in fact unconscious, with continued practice.

Gravity

Gravity plays a key role in stability ball exercises. As previously mentioned, balance is defined as effectively maintaining or moving one's center of gravity. Stability ball exercises involve moving the center of gravity in an unstable environment. Gravity is used in ball exercises to add resistance and increase the difficulty of a strengthening exercise or the effectiveness of a flexibility exercise. To use gravity effectively, one need only understand that as the body is positioned to work against gravity to greater and greater degrees, an exercise becomes more difficult. Consider performing a push-up on the stability ball. Lying prone over the ball with the ball under the abdomen requires the chest muscles to push a limited portion of body weight up against gravity. As one moves the ball further and further away from the abdomen, from under the pelvis to under the thighs to under the shins, more body weight is involved in the exercise (Figure 2.4). The chest muscles will work to push up progressively greater workloads against gravity, requiring greater muscle strength and increasing the challenge for the core muscles.

Positioning and Base Moves

Before performing exercises on the stability ball, it is critical that clients are able to balance, understand the basic movement positions, and are comfortable transitioning between moves. These things will assist exercisers in performing movements with good form and control. Finding balance through neutral spinal alignment is the first step (see Biomechanics, page 15). The following base positions need to be mastered before attempting exercises on the ball: the seated position, supine incline position, supine on floor with legs elevated, prone with trunk support position, side-lying position, and the supine bridge position (Ground Control Inc., 1995).

Seated Position

The seated position involves using the stability ball just like a chair. Instruct clients to sit upright on the center of the ball, positioned so that 90-degree angles are formed at both the

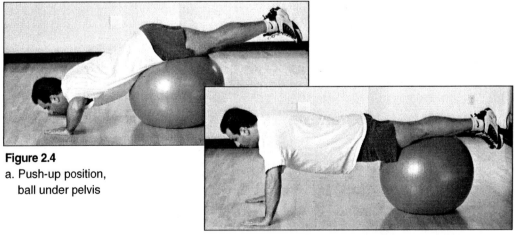

Figure 2.4
a. Push-up position, ball under pelvis

b. More challenging push-up position, ball under knees/upper shins

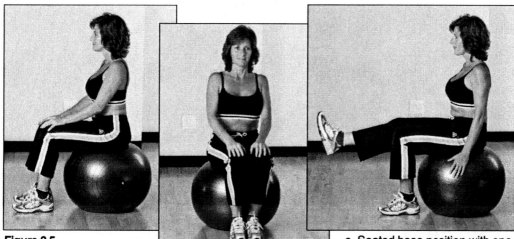

Figure 2.5

a. Seated base position

b. Seated base position with feet together for balance challenge

c. Seated base position with one leg lifted for greater balance challenge

knee and hip joints. Spinal alignment should be neutral and the back tall, chest lifted, and scapulae retracted. Arms should relax and hang naturally where most comfortable, while the feet are planted solidly on the floor shoulder-width apart and supporting little of the body weight (which is supported by the ball). From this base position, exercisers should be able to easily transition from one exercise position to another. Once they have mastered the seated base position, the balance challenge can be increased in a variety of ways (Figure 2.5). If the feet are positioned closer together than shoulder-width or one of the legs is lifted, requiring balance on only one foot while seated, a narrower base of support is created, which compromises balance and requires more effort to maintain proper positioning. Arm movements from any of these positions also add complexity and greater attention to balancing the center of gravity on the ball.

Supine Incline Position

The supine incline position requires the exerciser to lie back on the stability ball with neutral posture. The feet are firmly placed shoulder-width apart with a 90-degree angle at the knees. The ball is under the mid- and low-back area, supporting the torso in an inclined position (Figure 2.6). Clients should first be

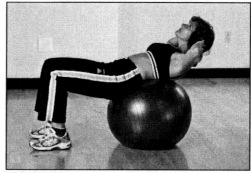

Figure 2.6
Supine incline base position

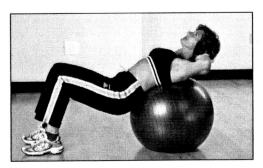

Figure 2.7
Modified supine incline base position, hips closer to the floor to create greater workload for quadriceps and glutes

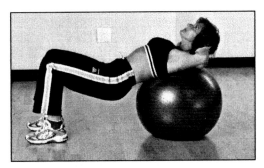

Figure 2.8
Hip flexor work; the pelvic tilt from supine incline base position

able to achieve this position with hands resting on the thighs, then while maintaining a neutral spine with the hands behind the head (providing light support) with elbows bent and open wide while keeping proper cervical alignment. Variations of the supine incline position involve adjusting the position of the spine over the ball. The more parallel to the floor the torso is, the greater the load displaced by the abdominal and neck muscles, while the load placed on the quadriceps and glutes is reduced. When the hips are closer to the floor and the torso is more inclined, the position creates less load on the abdominal and neck region and a greater load on the quadriceps and glutes (Figure 2.7). The ball should always be positioned so that the lower back is supported and is below the pivot point of the spine. Because the rectus abdominis is attached at the lower portion of the sternum and the pubis bone, the ball should not be placed above the rib cage if you want resistance to be placed on the abdominals. Also, if

the pelvis is allowed to move freely, such as when performing a pelvic tilt in the inclined position, the hip flexors, rather than the abdominals, are moving the joint (Figure 2.8). With the feet anchored on the floor and the upper torso anchored on the ball, there is no load resisting against spinal flexion. To effectively train the abdominals in this movement, de-anchor (lift) the lower body and anchor and stabilize the upper body and torso to move the lower region of the spine.

Supine on Floor with Legs Extended

The supine on floor with legs extended position places clients lying face up on the floor with the stability ball under the legs. Arms can rest on the floor, across the chest, or behind the head for increased challenge. The knees are flexed but slightly extended, and the calves or feet are hip-distance apart on the ball. As always, the spine should be neutral in this position (Figure 2.9). The farther the ball is from the hips, the greater the challenge

Figure 2.9
Supine with extended
legs base position

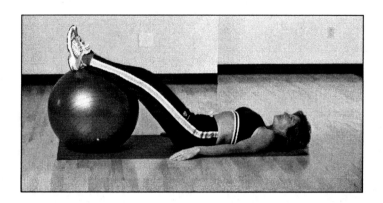

provided. Narrowing the distance between the feet or arms, or elevating one leg, also requires more effort to stabilize and balance the body. Variations on this base position are side-lying with elevated leg (Figure 2.10) and supine heel grip, where the legs and feet press into the ball, holding it firmly to the thighs.

Prone with Trunk Support

The prone with trunk support position is essentially resting on all fours with the ball under the torso. Instruct clients to kneel behind the ball, securing it against the knees, and lower the trunk to rest over the ball. Before

assuming this position, they should be taught transverse abdominis activation that involves contracting the abdomen to create intra-abdominal pressure, which protects the spine and low back while prone over the ball. Cue clients to "draw in" the abdomen, pulling the belly button toward the spine. Have them maintain this position throughout abdominal work while prone over the ball. Educate them to maintain normal breathing patterns while contracting the transverse abdominal muscle. Once prone over the ball, hands should rest on the floor, or on the ball for a greater challenge, with the body centered over the ball and the

Figure 2.10
Sidelying with
elevated leg
position

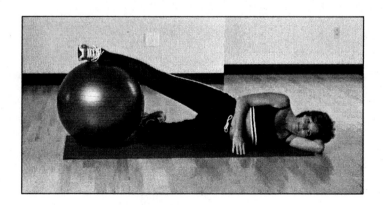

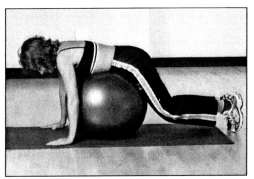

Figure 2.11
Prone with trunk support base position

spine neutral (Figure 2.11). If the size of the ball does not accommodate the length of the femur in this position, instruct clients to lift their knees off the floor until they can get their trunk parallel to the ground. Variations on this position that challenge the strength, balance, and coordination of the core muscles involve simply moving the ball farther away from the arms so it is centered under the pelvis and hips, under the thighs, or under the shins, with each variation requiring more work (Figure 2.12).

Side-lying

The side-lying base position can be performed with either a bent or straight leg, with the latter being a more challenging option. Exercisers kneel with the stability ball to one side, pressing against their hip. Direct them to lean into the ball and extend the leg farthest from the ball (the "top" leg) out to the side for balance. The leg closest to the ball can remain bent, providing a greater base of support for balance, or it can be extended and scissored in front or positioned behind the top leg for more challenge (Figure 2.13). Instruct them to maintain neutral spinal alignment at all times, especially in the cervical region, with the hip pressed firmly into the ball. Also, remind them to avoid allowing the hips to roll forward or back and to keep the shoulders aligned. Hands can be placed on the ball or, for increased support, the lower hand can extend to the floor.

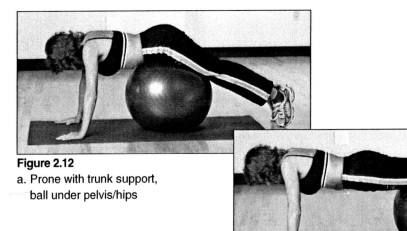

Figure 2.12
a. Prone with trunk support,
   ball under pelvis/hips

b. Prone with trunk support, ball under shins

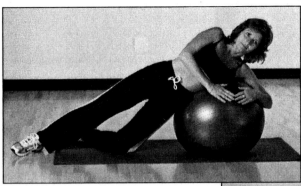

Figure 2.13
a. Side-lying base position with bent leg

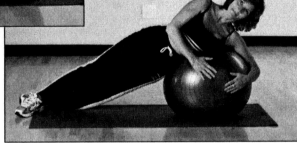

b. Side-lying base position with extended leg

Supine Bridge

The supine bridge position is sometimes referred to as supine with cervical support. To teach this position, have clients begin seated on the ball. They should roll down to a supine incline position and continue rolling until the head, shoulders, and upper back are resting on the ball, while the low back and hips are unsupported. Begin with the feet shoulder-width apart or wider and extend the hips and thighs parallel to the floor (forming a bridge), while keeping the knees flexed at 90 degrees and aligned over the heels (Figure 2.14). Balance can be further challenged by bringing the feet closer together or lifting one foot off the floor. It is critically important in this base position to have clients focus on the stabilizing muscles of the body, which for the supine bridge position are the quadriceps, hamstrings, glutes, and spinal extensors.

Figure 2.14
Supine bridge
base position

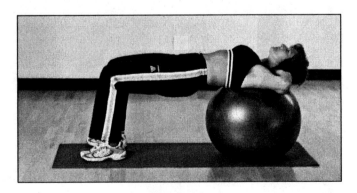

Transitioning

There are three steps that must be followed for exercisers to progress with safe and appropriate transitioning. Step one is to have them hold the base position while stabilizing the core and maintaining proper form and alignment. Once they can do this they can progress to step two, which involves adding the dynamic balance challenge of movement on, over, or around the ball, including working from positions with a decreased base of support. When adding external resistance, start with low resistance and progress appropriately.

While base positions are the starting and ending points for an exercise, proper cueing and execution are needed to transition from one base position or exercise to the next during a workout. Transitions can be very challenging, especially to novice ball users, older adults, and deconditioned, overweight, or balance-challenged individuals. In most cases, transitions involve walking: walking the legs out from the seated base position, walking the legs in from the supine incline position, walking with the hands from the prone position over the ball, and walking with the heels to move the ball away from or toward the thighs from the supine with elevated legs position.

There are several keys to transitioning smoothly and safely. Instruct clients to always take small steps to help maintain balance during movement when one foot or hand is lifted off the floor (or ball). Advise them to work to maintain neutral alignment in all portions of the spine during the transition. This is especially important for the cervical spine, as there is a tendency to lead with the head and neck when lifting from the ball, such as from supine incline to the seated position. For safety when lifting one leg off the floor, cue clients to begin with both hands on the floor for added stability. They can then progress to moving the hands onto the ball and finally resting on their body as the position allows. Have them execute all transitions in a slow and controlled manner, using the core stabilizers to maintain balance while moving.

Practicing transitions can be extremely helpful, especially for those newer to ball exercise who are unsure of the challenge different positions can provide. Allowing clients to "walk" back and forth between positions can help them determine which position will provide the most appropriate challenge to them for a particular exercise. For example, from the prone position over the ball, instruct clients to walk forward so the ball moves from under the torso to under the hips, thighs, and shins. Doing so will quickly and effectively provide them with feedback on the amount of torso stabilization and body strength required to maintain positions of varying degrees of difficulty. They can then be directed to select the position that meets their individual needs and goals based on the exercise being performed.

Programming

W hile the first three sections of this chapter (Workout Components, Cueing, and Music) are addressed specifically to group fitness instructors, the information can be applied to one-on-one training as well. It is important for personal trainers to understand how to design an effective warm-up and cool-down, as well as be able to safely lead exercisers through each individual movement. This chapter then moves into a discussion of proper progression and modifications, which are essential components of any stability ball workout.

Workout Components

Warm-up

As with any group fitness class, a stability ball workout should begin with an introduction followed by a few key questions. When working with a group, ask if any of the participants are in class for the first time and find out if this is their first experience with stability ball training. These questions are important so you know in advance which participants to watch even more carefully. Ask about the participants' health histories to determine whether any have had back, knee, or shoulder injuries or have a chronic condition such as hypertension. Again, these participants will need to be more closely monitored than others. They may need to be guided through certain exercises as well as presented options for exercises that are better suited to their condition (see Chapter Five).

Review the purpose of the stability ball class during the verbal introduction. Make participants aware of the focus of the class, such as strength training, flexibility training, or core training. Encourage them to pace themselves appropriately, to listen to their bodies at all times, and to select the version of each exercise that matches their fitness and experience levels. If there are some people who are new to ball training, a brief review of the benefits of ball training (posture, core strength, balance) also is recommended.

As with any workout, it is critical that a warm-up be provided in stability ball training. The goals of the warm-up are to increase body temperature and heart rate, increase synovial fluid production in the joints, and prepare the muscles for more vigorous movement. Depending on the format of the workout, the warm-up may need to be more vigorous (strength or core training) or less vigorous (flexibility or yoga training). In all cases, the length of the warm-up phase should run five to seven minutes depending on the fitness and experience level of the exercisers (longer for deconditioned individuals). Include a balanced blend of large rhythmic movements and dynamic stretches of major muscle groups that will be worked during the session. The warm-up can be designed as a traditional group exercise low-impact warm-up or may involve the use of the stability ball, which is recommended. During low-impact cardio-vascular movements, the ball can be held in the arms and moved in a variety of directions, which will familiarize exercisers with the size and shape of the ball and set a playful and fun tone for the workout. For a strength-training ball workout, the warm-up might include squats or lunges and range-of-motion upper-body movements near the ball, using it for support or to provide a reference point for movement depth. For a core-training session, the warm-up may take place from the seated position on the ball, including seated low-impact movements, hip circles and tilts, and movements to become familiar with the feeling of rolling the ball in different directions. At your discretion, the warm-up can be taught as a less vigorous, introductory version of the workout to come, and include large rhythmic movement patterns that prepare exercisers for the session. The warm-up also gives everyone a chance to learn and practice positions and exercises in a less intense, slower, controlled manner. For example, it might be an ideal time for teaching the six base positions.

Peak Training

Design the peak training section of a stability ball workout based on the goals and abilities of the exercisers. In general, focus on exercises to build muscle endurance, although muscle strength can also be worked by adding external resistance during some exercises or by adjusting body position on the ball. Include exercises to work every major muscle group. For muscle strengthening, eight to 12 repetitions per set are recommended for each exercise. For muscle endurance, the training guideline is 12 to 20 repetitions per set. Depending on the length of the session, one to three sets are advised. The goal is to overload the muscle or muscle groups significantly to produce fatigue and thereby muscle strength and/or endurance gains. Remind exercisers of this and urge them to rest or increase exercise difficulty as needed for their bodies.

For a flexibility-oriented workout, present stretches for every major muscle group in the body, with particular focus placed upon the muscles that tend to be tighter in most individuals (hip flexors, hamstrings, low back, and chest). For flexibility gains, hold each stretch for 30 seconds and repeat three to five times (American College of Sports Medicine, 2000). In a yoga workout, the positions will likely be held for 30 seconds to a minute and may or may not be repeated.

Cool-down

Lastly, all workouts require a cool-down segment, even flexibility and yoga. In this segment, core temperature should be reduced and the heart rate brought down to normal. Following a strength-training workout, the muscles worked will need to be stretched. If the session focused on flexibility, a different type of cool-down that incorporates relaxation and breathing can be used. The minimum length of the cool-down segment is three to five minutes.

Cueing

Giving appropriate and timely cues to participants is the cornerstone of group exercise. Classes including work on the stability ball are no different in that respect. In fact, cueing is one of the key factors for preventing injuries during stability ball work. First and foremost, communicate proper execution of an exercise, then demonstrate the starting position and movement. During the exercise demonstration, point out the most important aspects of correct body placement and purpose. Guide participants into the starting position for the exercise and give tips for proper technique. Explain which muscles to actively contract and where movement should come from (i.e., which joint, bone, or limb should move) and how far it should go. As participants begin executing the movement pattern, continue providing cues that encourage proper form for that particular exercise. For example, appropriate cues for abdominal oblique work would be "Make sure you have the feet slightly staggered and knees slightly rotated to one side" and "As you lift and contract, drive the base of the ribcage toward the hip." Watch the participants' form during ball work and explain what to avoid doing as well. For example, "Make sure to keep the pelvis stable in neutral posture" is a common cue in many exercises.

Cue participants through different options for a particular exercise, as they may need more or less of a challenge. When doing so, guide them to listen to their own bodies and select the appropriate level for their abilities and needs. Give ample encouragement to participants at all levels, with special attention provided to newcomers and novice stability ball users. Tell advanced participants to adjust from the more challenging position when they feel their form being compromised by fatigue. For example, when performing a bench press, participants might start from the supine position. Once they have reached the point of fatigue, adjust the position to the supine bridge position, which offers support for the shoulder girdle and requires less shoulder stabilization. This change in position will allow the participant to achieve a few more repetitions prior to momentary muscle failure without increasing their risk of injury.

Music

Select music according to the pace and types of exercises being performed. For muscle strength and endurance work, core-training exercises, and balance training, the appropriate music speed ranges from 110 to 130 beats per minute (bpm). Music speed above 130 bpm can affect the ability to move in a slow and controlled manner, allowing momentum to play a role in exercise execution and reducing the effectiveness and safety of ball exercises. Also consider the preferences and tastes of the exercisers.

Flexibility exercises performed on the stability ball require softer, somewhat relaxing music choices. Movements are not performed in cadence to a beat, so relaxation music is fitting. Depending on the overall workout design, however, if ball stretches are incorporated into the strength work rather than used as a cool-down, the music guidelines described previously are appropriate.

Techniques and Proper Progression

There are a number of techniques for adjusting the intensity of an exercise on the stability ball. In Chapter Two, the section on Balance (page 12) reviewed ways to increase and decrease the amount of balance required to hold a position on the stability ball. A wider base of support with either a greater portion of the body or more limbs in contact with the floor creates a less challenging situation for the exerciser. Balance can be challenged with as small a move as changing from a flat foot on the floor to one that is dorsiflexed so only the heel touches the ground. Essentially, less contact with the floor requires more balance on the rounded surface of the ball, which challenges exercisers to greater and greater degrees.

Intensity can also be altered by changing the position of the ball under or over the body, which often involves moving the body into a different position against gravity. Moving greater portions of the body against gravity creates greater resistance. Consider supine hip extension to work the gluteus maximus and hamstrings. The easiest position starts from the supine on floor with legs extended base position, where the torso rests on the floor with the ball under the legs, knees are flexed, and the ball presses against the thighs and calves. In this exercise, the hips are extended slowly and the hamstrings and glutes tighten to contract the pelvis up against gravity and create an aligned body from knees to shoulders (Figure 3.1 a & b). To vary the intensity of this exercise, move the ball away from the thighs so the starting position involves less knee flexion and just the calves and feet rest on the ball. For even greater difficulty, extend the knees further so only

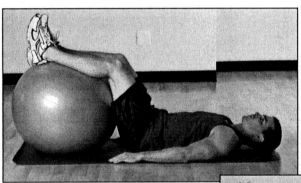

Figure 3.1
a. Supine hip extension start position for gluteus maximus and hamstrings

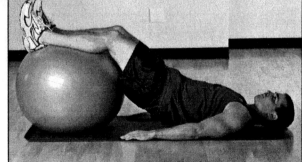

b. End position

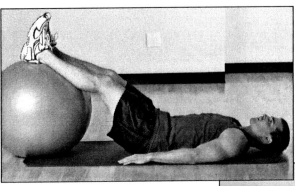

Figure 3.1 (continued)
c. Start position for more intense supine hip extension work, ball under calves

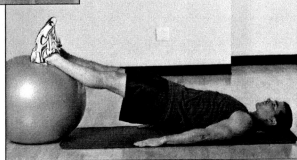

d. End position

the heels contact the ball (Figure 3.1 c & d). Both of these variations involve a greater amount of body weight being lifted against gravity to perform the exercise (in addition to creating a greater balance challenge with less of the body in contact with the ball). To further increase the resistance and balance challenge, one leg can be elevated. This causes the support side of the body to work harder to perform hip extension as hip rotator and oblique muscles work to help stabilize the body.

Another creative technique for altering the challenge provided by stability ball exercises is to vary the timing of an exercise, the number of repetitions, or the speed of movement. All of these variables should be adjusted according to the goals and abilities of each exerciser. Increasing the

number of repetitions adds challenge to a movement, as does moving more slowly. Varying the timing of an exercise also adds variety to the routine, such as changing from a two-counts-up, two-counts-down cadence to a three-counts-up, one-count-down pattern. This provides a greater challenge, as exercisers have to work longer during the more difficult phase of a movement. For example, during the traditional crunch exercise with the ball positioned under the middle to lower back and hips, greater work is required of the upper portion of the rectus abdominis muscle. Changing the timing pattern of the basic crunch so they move one count up and three counts down requires exercisers to spend more time in the eccentric phase of the abdominal contraction, working more against gravity and providing much more challenge. The best timing or speed of movement is one that can be fully controlled. Watch that clients avoid using momentum to perform the ball exercises. If the speed is too fast for them, it is more likely that they will use momentum rather than controlled, deliberate movements.

When varying exercise intensity and designing the stability ball exercise routine for a class, the number one issue to consider is the audience. Ask yourself a variety of questions about the make-up of your class when putting together the routine of ball exercises for a group. Who is participating in the class? Are most of the exercisers very fit individuals who can safely perform advanced exercises? Or are they novice stability ball users who are deconditioned? Are there any special populations in the class that will require extra attention such as pre- and post-natal women, older adults, children, or very heavy individuals? By thinking through these questions, you will be prepared to offer a variety of exercise options to meet the needs of most, if not all, participants, so that everyone in class gets a safe and effective stability ball workout.

Modifications

I t is extremely important that you are knowledgeable about the appropriate ways to modify a stability ball exercise to meet the variety of needs of each exerciser. Clear understanding of the use of the techniques described previously is required. In all cases

where an exercise beyond a base move is shown, you must be able to cue exercisers back to the base move if they are adversely challenged. This may be observed when someone cannot maintain correct posture and alignment to perform the exercise. If form is compromised, it is critical that you be able to provide a less-challenging option. To do so, you can direct exercisers to increase their contact with the floor, creating a greater base of support so balance is less challenged. For example, during supine incline oblique curls, if an exerciser cannot balance enough (with feet wide on the floor and hands behind the head) to twist the torso effectively, cue him or her to place the fingertips of the opposite hand on the floor for support (Figure 3.2).

Another way to modify a ball exercise is to adjust the position on the ball. The closer the stability ball is to the pivot point of movement,

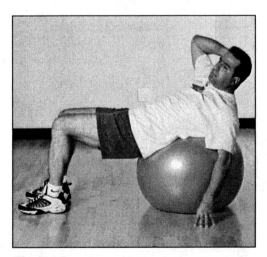

Figure 3.2
Modified supine incline oblique curls, fingers on floor to decrease balance challenge

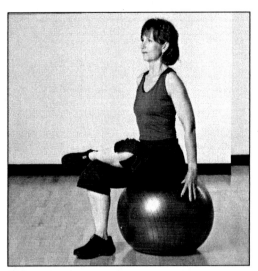

Figure 3.3
Seated hip/glute stretch

example, consider the seated outer thigh (hip/glute) stretch on the ball. Have exercisers maintain a neutral spine in the seated position with both feet flat on the floor. The ankle of one leg is then crossed over the thigh of the other, which remains in contact with the ground (Figure 3.3). This may be too challenging a stretch for some due to the balance challenge created, while it may be too easy for others. Modifications to this stretch involve moving the base leg farther away from the ball and emphasizing a slight anterior tilt of the pelvis (this is an easier stretch for the hip/glute) and dorsiflexing the base foot so only the heel rests on the floor (providing greater balance challenge) (Figure 3.4). You can also direct clients to keep the foot of the base leg flat on the ground and lean forward for a greater hip stretch, changing the center of gravity over the ball and again

the easier the exercise becomes. For example, if an exerciser has trouble correctly performing push-ups from the prone position with the ball under the hips, direct him or her to move the ball closer to the center of movement (the chest) by moving the ball under the lower or middle abdomen. Remember that most of the exercises performed on the stability ball can be performed off the ball in a modified way. If a client is showing signs of fatigue and the inability to properly execute the least challenging option for an exercise on the ball, consider eliminating the ball from that exercise. In the push-up example above, should the exerciser still be unable to perform the movement correctly, have him or her perform push-ups off the ball and then return to the ball for the next exercise.

Small adjustments in body position are often all that is required to help exercisers get an effective stretch on the ball as well. For

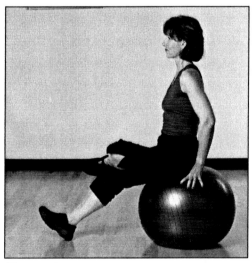

Figure 3.4
Modified seated hip/glute stretch, base leg extended and foot dorsiflexed for less hip/glute stretch and greater balance challenge

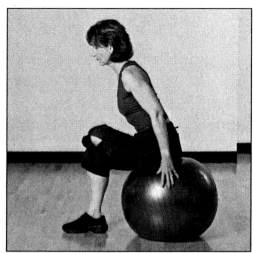

Figure 3.5
Modified hip/glute stretch, forward lean for increased hip/glute stretch and greater balance challenge

challenging balance (Figure 3.5). Another way to begin this exercise is with the ball positioned within arm's reach from a wall in the room, so everyone can perform the exercise at an appropriate intensity with less of a balance challenge. For deconditioned individuals, the ball can be placed against the wall or the stretch can be performed from the supine on floor with legs extended position. Both modifications yield much less of a balance challenge.

You can also modify strength exercises by adjusting the amount and/or type of resistance utilized or by changing the position of the body on the ball to create greater opposition to the force of gravity. If an exerciser is unable to maintain proper form and balance on the ball while performing shoulder raises from the seated position with 8-pound weights, have him or her decrease the weight lifted. If this adjustment is made and he or she is still unable to maintain proper spinal alignment and hold a safe, neutral position on the ball, tell him or her to lower the weight more or perform the exercises without any added resistance. Even though making the movement a body-weight exercise will provide less local muscle challenge, it will train the core musculature for posture and balance. This will establish neuro-muscular movement patterns that train him or her to perform the exercise correctly with added resistance in the future.

Stretches can be adjusted with the addition of a towel or non-elastic stretch strap. For example, a towel can be used to enhance a triceps stretch from the seated position on the ball (Figure 3.6).

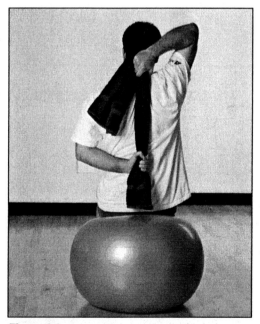

Figure 3.6
Modified triceps stretch (using towel) from seated base position

Injury Prevention

The critical issues to preventing injuries during stability ball work include proper exercise progression and self-monitoring by the exerciser. In a class setting, proper cueing and careful observation on the part of the instructor are also essential. As previously mentioned, you must have a thorough understanding of biomechanics and body alignment when teaching ball exercises, and be able to effectively communicate those issues for each exercise. It is also important that you know what movements or position variations need to be avoided for each exerciser to accommodate their individual fitness levels. Be prepared to explain why those moves or positions are contraindicated and make corrections and teach modifications for each person's unique body size and needs.

High-risk and Contraindicated Movements

With stability ball exercises, many of the advanced options can be "high-risk" for certain people. Individuals with little or no ability to balance their bodies on the balls, control their body weights against gravity, or maintain neutral spinal alignment in an exercise should be provided with and encouraged to perform alternative, less challenging exercises. More intense versions of an exercise on the ball should only be attempted by those who have demonstrated mastery of the basic principles of stability ball use (balance and proper form during transitions and at least the less intense variations of an exercise). Progress exercisers gradually and appropriately toward increased challenges. While some ball exercises are high-risk for certain populations (see Chapter Five), other movements are contraindicated for everyone.

Fast, ballistic movements on the stability ball are discouraged unless they come during the cardio warm-up or cool-down of a ball class. However, even the faster movements performed in these situations should be done in a controlled, deliberate manner. The lack of control often associated with fast movements allows momentum to play a larger role in movement than muscle contraction, as well as causes an even greater balance challenge that many exercisers cannot tolerate. Additionally, movements that hyperflex or hyperextend a joint, forcing it beyond its normal range of motion, are contraindicated. For example, the supine incline base position involves reclining on the ball with the feet hip-distance apart on the floor. In this position, the knees are flexed to a 90-degree angle. As exercisers become fatigued in the core, they tend to sink the glutes toward the floor and make the body less horizontal. Watch for and correct hyperflexion of the knees, which occurs when this position is done without moving the feet away from the ball to keep the 90-degree angle at the knees (Figure 3.7).

The stability ball supports the body weight, which reduces pressure and shearing force on the

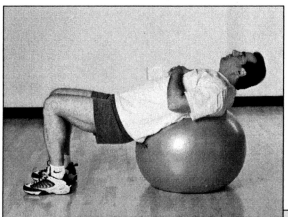

Figure 3.7
a. Supine incline base position with proper 90-degree knee flexion

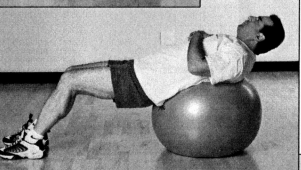

b. Supine incline base position with acceptable knee flexion (greater than 90 degrees)

c. Unacceptable supine incline base position (knees flexed to less than 90-degree angle)

knee. This makes deep knee flexion significantly less risky on the ball than in a standing deep squat. However, for some people it is still a risky movement that can cause knee discomfort. It is recommended that knee flexion beyond 90 degrees be generally avoided for extended periods of time, such as when holding a position to train the abdominals. Special exceptions are allowed for yoga and flexibility movements using the stability ball that involve holding a position for a limited amount of time and performing moves in a very controlled manner with constant focus on body position specifically to feel a stretch in a particular muscle or muscle group (and offering options for participants that cannot flex the knees as a position dictates).

Types of Stability Ball Programs

CHAPTER FOUR

Strength Training on the Ball

Most of the strength-training exercises typically done in a group fitness class or personal training session can be done in a similar way with the stability ball. When incorporating resistance equipment, such as free weights, tubing, or weighted bars, into stability ball work, focus on developing muscle endurance rather than strength. Note that barbells are not recommended. Muscle-endurance training focuses on the number of times a muscle can exert force against a submaximal resistance, while muscle-strength training focuses on the maximal amount of force a muscle or muscle group can exert against a resistance. The core work required of the torso during ball training is an example of endurance work, requiring the postural muscles to maintain neutral spinal alignment at all times. When designing a workout, focus on high repetitions with moderate resistance (muscle-endurance training guidelines) rather than low repetitions with maximal resistance (muscle-strength training guidelines). That is not to say that an exercise designed for endurance training will not actually be muscle-strength training for some people, especially those that are newer to exercise, new to ball training, or new to strength training. However, clients should use lighter resistance when performing stability ball work than they normally would when strength training.

The most important issue related to strength training on the ball is safety. Proper body positioning and control are required for each exercise and should be of the utmost concern. If exercisers are unable to support themselves with proper form, advise them to adjust their position on the ball to one that is less challenging, especially if they are performing an exercise that uses an additional piece of strength-training equipment. In addition, clients should reduce the amount of resistance or terminate an exercise if fatigued to avoid injury. It is critical that you have a thorough understanding of biomechanics and proper body alignment for each strength-training

exercise attempted on the ball. This will ensure exercises performed are not only safe and effective, but also best able to meet the goals of each exerciser. Because quick assessment is not always possible in a group fitness setting, advise participants to first use low resistance until you are comfortable with their technique.

The skill or ability level and fitness goals of each person will determine several important things for strength training on the ball. First is the amount of control they are capable of maintaining during an exercise. Newer or deconditioned exercisers, as well as those with poor balance such as many older adults or overweight individuals, will have more trouble maintaining body control while exercising on the ball. Range of motion is also determined by the needs of each exerciser. Individuals who find it challenging to control their body weight on the ball may need to perform strength-training exercises with a somewhat limited range of motion and less resistance challenge, as should those recovering from bone, muscle, or joint injuries. Advise individuals seeking muscle-strength gains, and those with significant exercise and strength-training experience, to select somewhat heavier weights or perform the more challenging version of a particular movement pattern. However, remind them that the goal when combining resistance equipment with stability ball training should be improving muscle endurance while simultaneously enhancing stabilization and neuromuscular efficiency. Also, only recommend muscle-strength training if an exerciser can maintain proper spinal alignment and correct form in the easier version of the exercise with lighter weights. Proper exercise progression is the key factor for everyone.

The sample exercises below review, through photos and brief descriptions, one strength exercise for each major muscle group using the stability ball (Figures 4.1 through 4.12).

Each workout should begin with a cardio warm-up and dynamic stretches and end with a cool-down, including stretches to improve flexibility. The exercises are presented in an order that most easily allows for transitions between exercise positions so that the session or class flows smoothly.

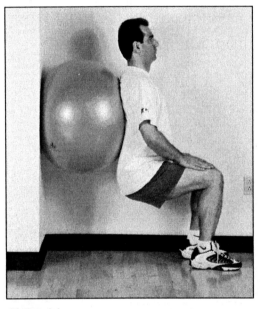

Figure 4.1
Wall squat with ball behind back

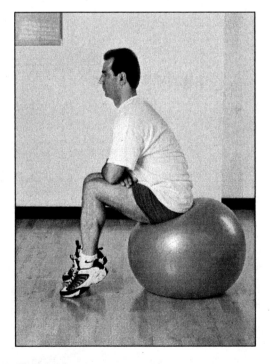

Figure 4.2
Seated calf raises on the ball

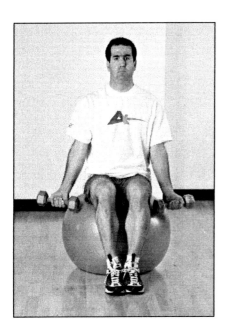 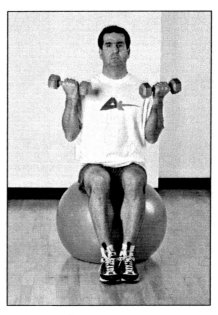

Figure 4.3
Seated bicep curls on the ball

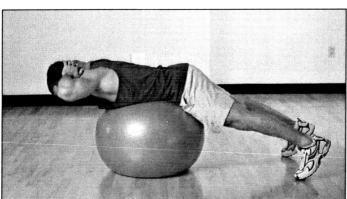

Figure 4.4
Prone over the ball back (trunk) extensions

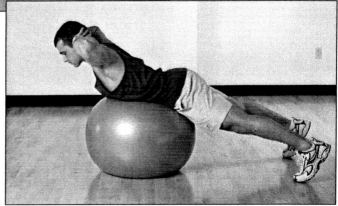

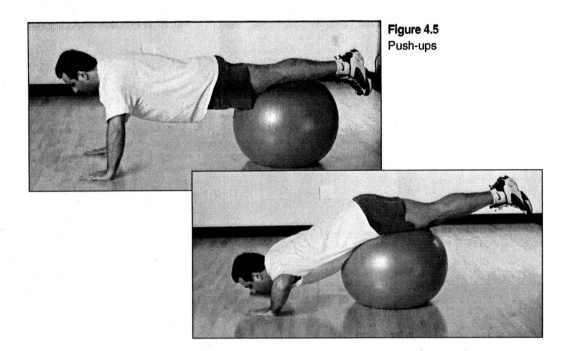

Figure 4.5
Push-ups

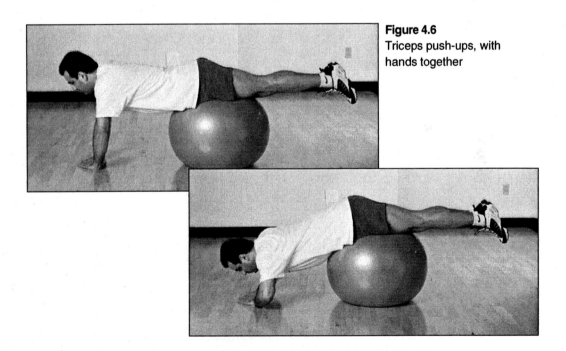

Figure 4.6
Triceps push-ups, with hands together

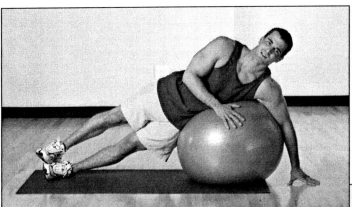

Figure 4.7
Side-lying hip abduction

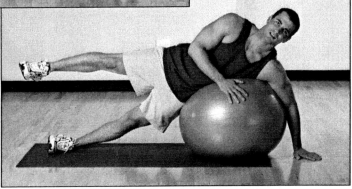

Figure 4.8
Side-lying oblique curls

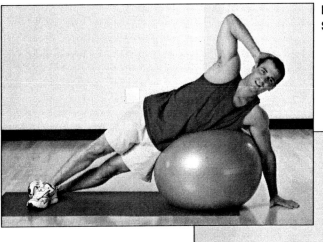

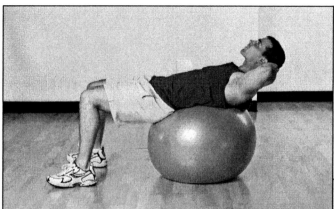

Figure 4.9
Abdominal crunches on the ball
for rectus abdominis (supine
incline trunk curl)

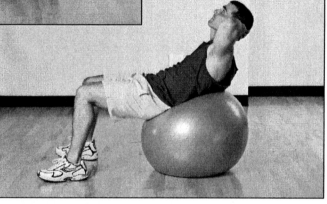

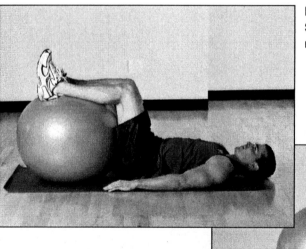

Figure 4.10
Supine with elevated legs
reverse curls

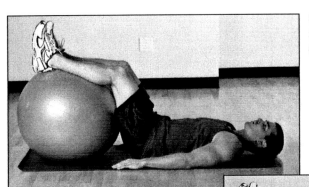

Figure 4.11
Supine with elevated legs
hip extension

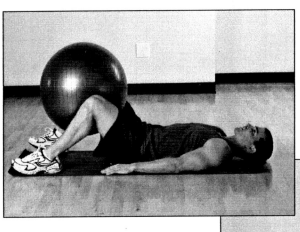

Figure 4.12
a. Hip adduction, ball
   between thighs/knees

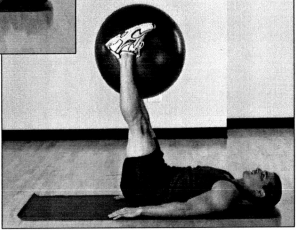

b. Hip adduction, ball between calves/ankles

Incorporating Equipment

The ball is the primary base of support for all strength-training exercises that use equipment. Because it is an unstable base of support, that in itself is a challenge. Added equipment provides extra resistance, but should only be used once exercisers have appropriately mastered the basic ball positions and can maintain body alignment through core stabilization for extended periods of time.

Free weights can be used to strength train on the ball, providing either bilateral or unilateral resistance. Upper-body strength-training exercises can be performed from the seated base position, including biceps, triceps, deltoid, and back work (Figure 4.13). Chest, anterior deltoid, and triceps work with weights can be accomplished from the supine incline and bridge positions (Figure 4.14). From the supine incline position, the ball is placed under the back, supporting the core, and the shoulders are not

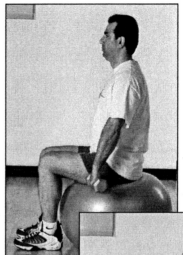

Figure 4.13
Anterior deltoid work with free weights, from the seated base position

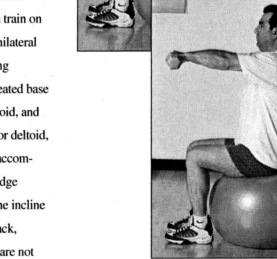

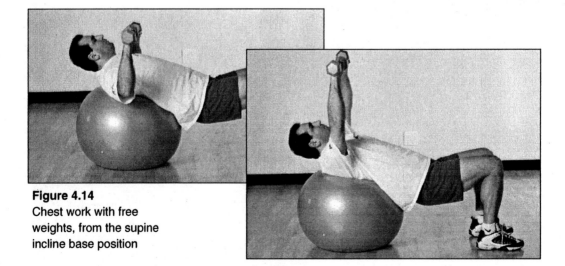

Figure 4.14
Chest work with free weights, from the supine incline base position

45

supported. With added resistance, more shoulder stabilization is required, making the chest work more challenging. This is also a challenging position for the neck as it is unsupported by the ball. In the bridge position, the ball rests under the cervical spine, providing support to the shoulders, while the lower body maintains a bridge position with the torso and thighs parallel to the floor, and the knees bent at 90 degrees. Stabilization comes from the mid-back muscles, erector spinae, glutes, hamstrings, hip abductors and adductors, and legs. As the shoulders are supported by the ball, less shoulder stabilization is required to work the chest, making the movements less challenging (however, more stabilization is required by the rest of the body, which can be very challenging).

While prone over the ball at the base position, upper- and mid-back work (also posterior deltoid, biceps, and shoulder work) can be performed with free weights. Note the need for a neutral neck in this position (Figure 4.15). Additional shoulder work, as well as hip work, can be performed from the side-lying position. Performing any of the bilateral exercises here with only one arm will increase the difficulty of maintaining balance on the ball. The moving limb alters the center of gravity greatly, while bilateral work shifts the center of gravity evenly with less of a balance challenge.

A lightly weighted bar can be used in place of free weights to perform much of the strength work described here, requiring the arms to work simultaneously with a two-handed grip (Figure 4.16).

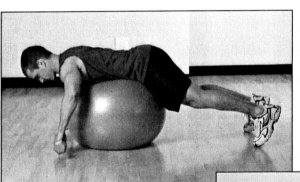

Figure 4.15
Upper- and mid-back work with free weights, from the prone over the ball base position

Additional exercises that can be performed with the weighted bar involve using the bar as a prop to provide balance (resting the bar vertically with one end on the floor). From the seated or supine incline base positions the bar helps clients balance to perform one-legged squats (Figure 4.17) or during the bridge with one leg lifted off the floor.

Elastic resistance, such as bands or tubes, is also effective for strength training on the stability ball. Weighted equipment challenges exercisers to move the weight against gravity. Therefore, to make the strength work most effective, the body and free weight need to be positioned so that the working muscle contracts in the direction opposite

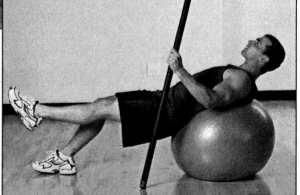

Figure 4.16
Anterior deltoid work with a weighted bar, from the seated base position

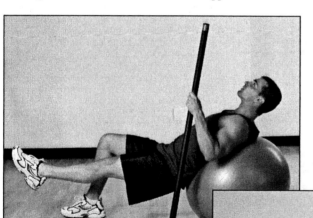

Figure 4.17
One-legged squat from the supine incline base position using a weighted bar for balance support

gravity. Elastic resistance, however, allows the direction of muscle pull to be anywhere. As the tube is pulled from a central or anchored point, it stretches, and the resistance the muscle must overcome to perform the movement increases. Strength training with elastic resistance trains for muscle endurance and allows for great variety in body placement when performing muscle-strength work. Exercises can be performed from the seated base position, supine incline, and bridge (Figures 4.18 through 4.20).

Figure 4.18
Upright row with elastic resistance, from the seated base position

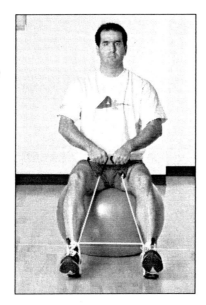 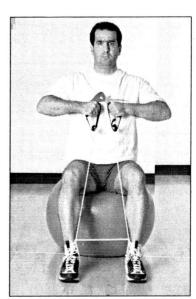

Figure 4.19
Upper- and mid-back work with elastic resistance, from the seated base position

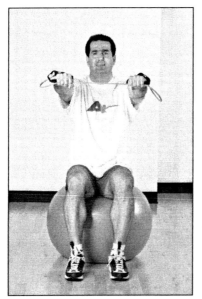 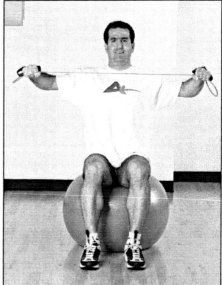

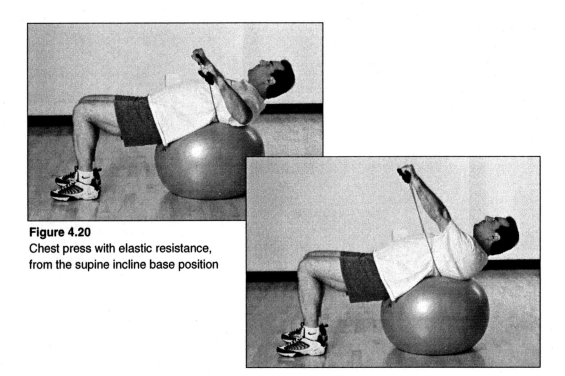

Figure 4.20
Chest press with elastic resistance, from the supine incline base position

Flexibility Training on the Ball

The stability ball is one of the most versatile and effective tools for improving flexibility. The ball can be used to enhance traditional passive stretches by allowing for a greater range of motion than can be normally achieved (e.g., the seated lateral torso stretch on the ball allows for a greater stretch by repositioning the hips by rolling the ball). The ball also facilitates active stretches, where one muscle or muscle group is stretching while the opposing muscle(s) and/or stabilizing muscles are contracting, such as during an active hamstring stretch seated on the ball. As the leg is extended to stretch the hamstring, the quadriceps muscles contract to hold the leg in an elevated position, while the core musculature contracts to stabilize the body in position for the stretch. Lastly, the stability ball can be used to perform dynamic stretches, where movement of the ball is used to provide, deepen, or add challenge to a stretch. For example, hip circles from the seated position promote dynamic lumbar spine mobility. Another example of dynamic stretching with the ball is the supine shoulder stretch. Here the exerciser rests supine on the floor holding the ball in his or her hands with the arms extended toward the ceiling. To stretch, he or she slowly lowers the ball toward the floor on one side of the body, arms moving in horizontal abduction and adduction, to stretch the deltoid of the arm

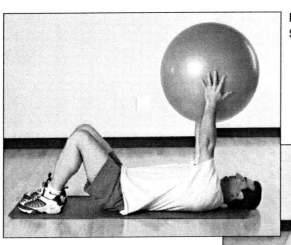

Figure 4.21
Supine shoulder stretch

closer to the ceiling (Figure 4.21). Other examples of dynamic stretching are found in yoga training on the stability ball.

Flexibility training and strength training on the ball are similar in that the spinal stabilizers and core musculature are working to maintain posture at all times. Balance and coordination are also utilized during flexibility training on the ball, similar to strength training. Other benefits of flexibility training with a stability ball include comfort and ease of use. For many exercisers, it is preferable to be off the floor, especially for older adults and overweight individuals who have trouble getting down to and up from the ground. In terms of ease of use, the stability ball provides smooth progressions as exercisers gently roll from one position to the next. Transitions between movements can be more rhythmic because of the

ball's dynamic structure, which also supports the body. The ball allows exercisers to achieve positions that elongate the spine, reduce compression, and encourage the spinal muscles to relax. Its curved shape allows for certain stretches that are not possible on the floor. Stretching on the ball is also time-efficient, as endurance is developed in certain muscles while training for flexibility in others. Lastly, flexibility training is simply more fun on the ball for many exercisers. Those who usually skip the flexibility portion of their exercise routine might find the ball more entertaining and playful, increasing their interest and improving the likelihood of actually performing stretches regularly.

Guidelines for designing a flexibility-training program on the stability ball are similar to those for strength training. Controlling the movement is extremely important for injury prevention, and here, too, your knowledge of biomechanics will help with effective exercise design and execution. Monitor range of motion to avoid over-stretching, and target muscle groups according to individual needs. Options for limited range of motion need to be presented to accommodate exercisers of varying levels of flexibility and strength, with an emphasis on paying attention to the body's signals about how a stretch feels. Have exercisers progress slowly and with control at all times, and cue them to breathe normally, as many people have a tendency to hold the breath when stretching. Demonstrate how to come out of a stretch, and make them feel comfortable doing so at any time should they experience discomfort in any stretch position.

Stretching on the stability ball, as with any stretching, should not be performed until a thorough warm-up of at least five minutes has been completed. Once done, stretch all major muscle groups with at least three to five sets per muscle group. When executing a stretch, hold for a minimum of 30 seconds to achieve maximal flexibility gains with minimal chance or injury. Have exercisers "ride the edge of a stretch" so they are pushing a muscle or muscle group to the point of mild tension without experiencing pain. Make position adjustments as flexibility improves to gradually progress to greater ranges of motion. For greater flexibility gains, stretching can be performed when muscles are relaxed (in addition to warm), as this will promote

lengthening of the muscle fibers. All stretches should be performed slowly and with total control to avoid injury.

Proper body alignment is crucial and needs to be monitored at all times during a stability ball workout. Select stretches that allow exercisers the greatest opportunity to make flexibility gains, and involve positions appropriate to their skills and ability levels with the ball so they are not at undue risk for injury. Take advantage of the unique opportunity the ball provides to stretch muscles in a wide variety of positions with numerous exercise variations, rather than performing the same stretches all the time. This will help everyone achieve greater improvements in both active and passive flexibility. For example, to actively stretch the hamstrings from the seated position, the exerciser contracts the opposing muscle group (the quadriceps) (Figure 4.22). The same muscle group can be stretched

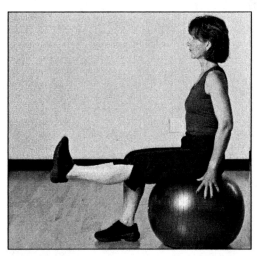

Figure 4.22
Active stretch of the hamstrings from the seated base position

passively, as shown in Figure 4.23. In both positions the core muscles isometrically contract to stabilize and assist balance on the ball. The ball is therefore uniquely time-efficient and functional as exercisers are simultaneously developing both active and passive flexibility and muscle endurance. These gains in turn lead to improved functional fitness in daily activities, decreased risk of injury, and less muscle soreness from both daily activities and cardiovascular and strength exercise.

The following sample stretches provide an example of one stretch for most major muscle groups. Stretches are presented for beginner-level exercisers and are designed in an order that minimizes position changes (Figures 4.24 through 4.34).

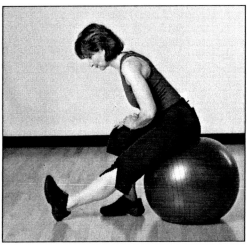

Figure 4.23
Passive hamstring stretch from the seated base position

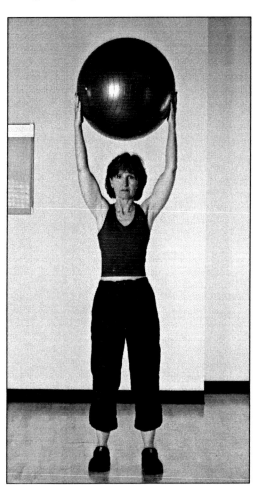

Figure 4.24
Standing shoulder stretch

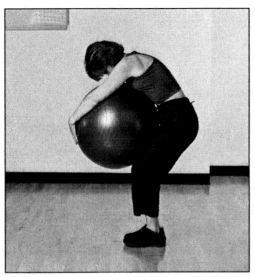
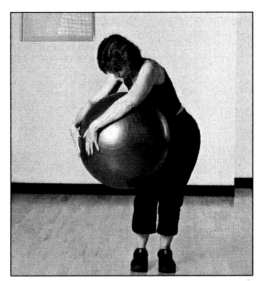

Figure 4.25
Standing back stretch with ball on thighs and rotary torso movement

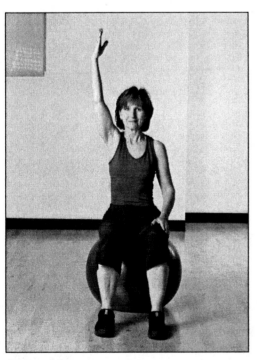
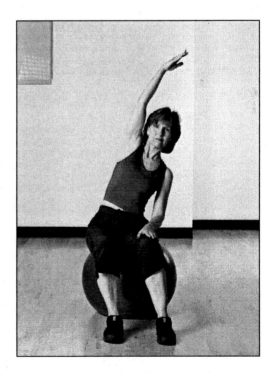

Figure 4.26
Seated lateral torso (trunk) stretch

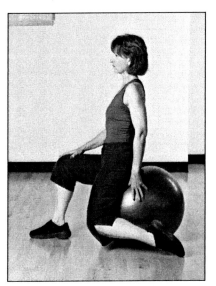

Figure 4.27
Seated hip flexor/quadriceps/anterior
tibialis stretch

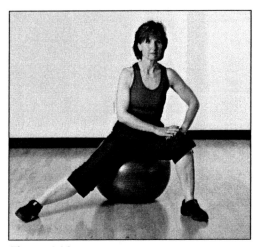

Figure 4.28
Seated adductor
stretch (lunge)

Figure 4.29
Supine incline
hip/glute stretch

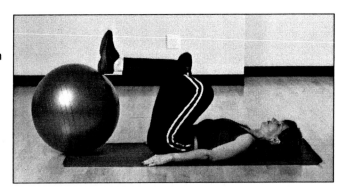

Figure 4.30
Supine Incline
spinal traction

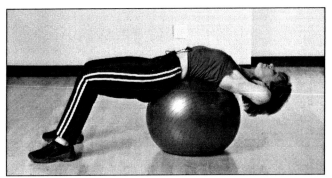

Figure 4.31
Prone kneeling chest/anterior shoulder stretch

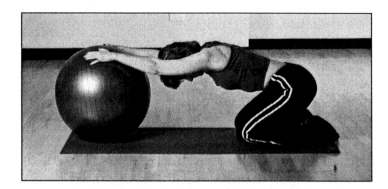

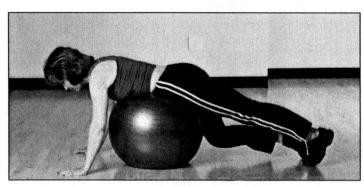

Figure 4.32
Prone calf/soleus stretch

Figure 4.33
Supine with elevated legs torso stretch (with rotary torso movement)

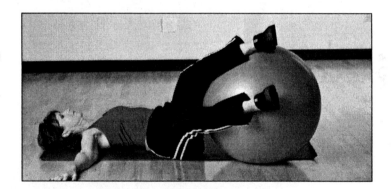

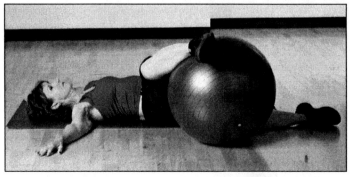

Figure 4.34
Supine with elevated legs scissor stretch

Mind/Body Exercise

One of the more recent trends in fitness involves using the ball with mind-body modalities such as yoga and Pilates. The stability ball works to help exercisers add challenge with its active balance component. Or, alternatively, the ball can be used to provide support in more challenging exercises for those not quite up to the skill or strength level needed for a particular movement. For example, two poses where the stability ball can be helpful to yoga instructors are the plank, and the downward facing dog (Figures 4.35 and 4.36). Challenge can be added with the ball in other poses, such as the bridge (Figure 4.37).

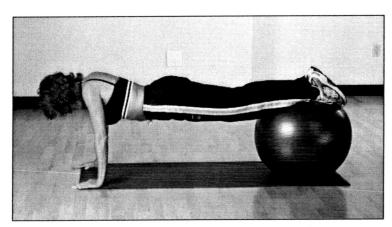

Figure 4.35
Plank position with and without the ball

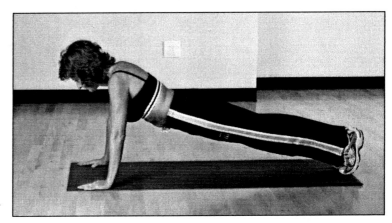

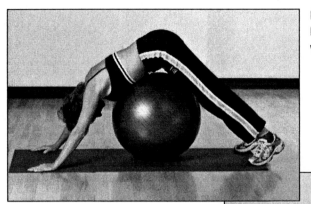

Figure 4.36
Downward facing dog with and without the ball

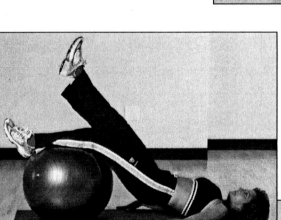

Figure 4.37
Bridge position with and without the ball

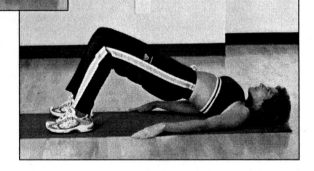

Core Training and Balance

Training the core musculature is one of the primary uses of the stability ball. There is a wide variety of exercises to train the abdominal and back muscles. Additionally, there are ways to train balance with the ball both alone and simultaneously while muscle strength or endurance training. The exercises presented here are meant to provide a basic understanding of stability ball use for core and balance training and can be incorporated into any ball class or workout. For any of the balance exercises presented, instruct exercisers to stay within an arm's length of a wall or chair for support should the exercises be too challenging. Workouts can be designed to work only balance and core muscles as well, incorporating the principles used in the exercises presented on the following pages (Figures 4.38 through 4.48).

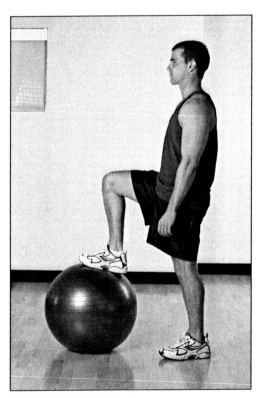

Figure 4.38
Standing one-leg balance

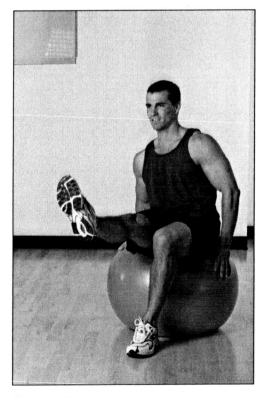

Figure 4.39
Seated one-leg balance

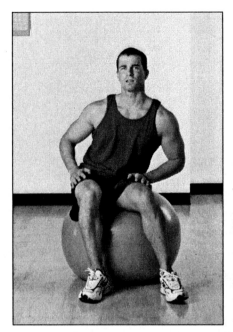
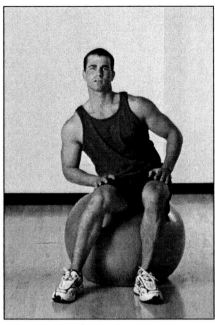

Figure 4.40
Seated lumbar mobility (hip circles and pelvic tilts)

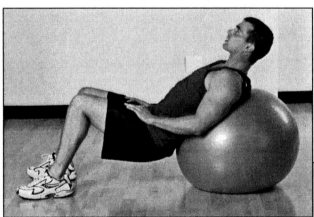

Figure 4.41
Supine incline pelvic tilt

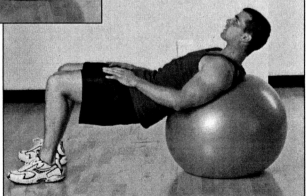

Figure 4.42
Supine incline/parallel trunk curl

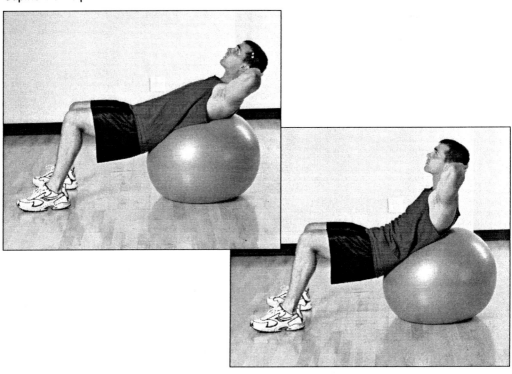

Figure 4.43
a. Supine incline oblique curl

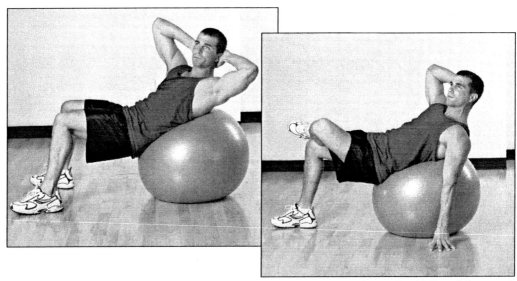

b. Cross leg option for supine incline oblique curl, with hand on floor for assistance

Figure 4.44

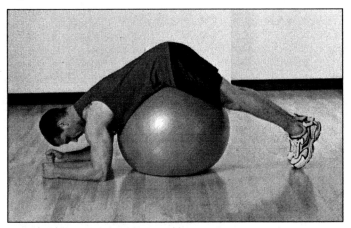

a. Prone hip extension start position

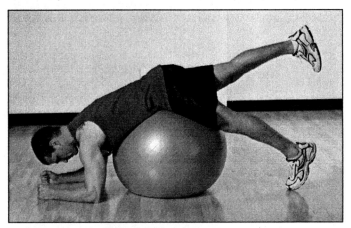

b. Prone hip extension one leg option

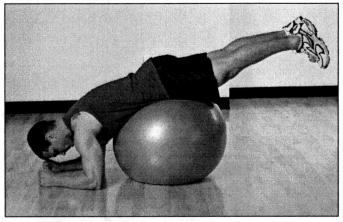

c. Prone hip extension both legs option

Figure 4.45
Prone trunk extension

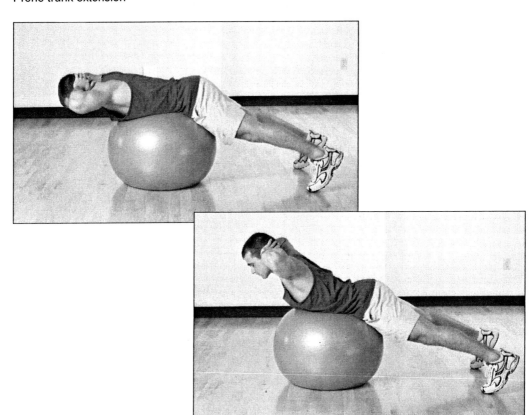

Figure 4.46
Prone opposite arm/opposite leg raise

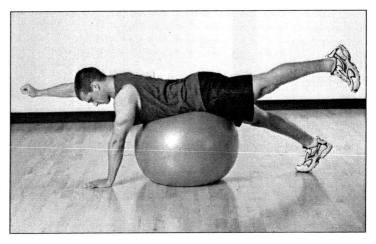

Figure 4.47
a. Rolling lat pull start position, arms extended

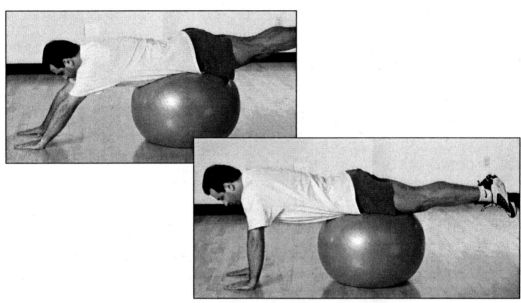

b. Ending position, wrists under shoulders

Figure 4.48
Supine with elevated legs reverse curl

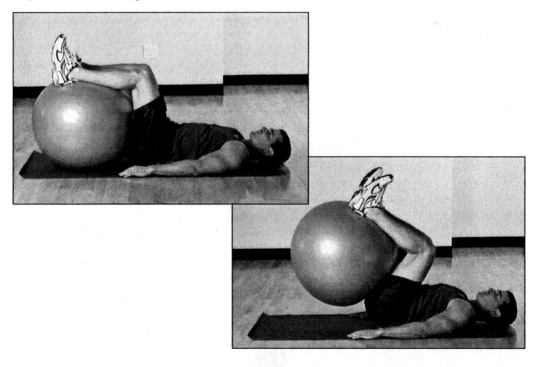

Integrating the Stability Ball into Other Group Fitness Classes

Even if a facility is unable to provide scheduled times for a "stability ball class," the ball can still be used. With its myriad benefits, ball use is highly recommended for integration into portions of other classes where it can be used for short periods of time to strengthen or stretch specific muscle groups. For example, the ball might be used during the final cool-down of a step class to perform stretches for all the major muscle groups. The stability ball can also be used to perform core work toward the end of a low-impact class, or included for use with certain exercises during a muscle-conditioning class, along with other forms of

resistance. Circuit training and "boot camp" classes can also involve the ball simply by using it as one of many "stations" participants work through. Lastly, the stability ball can be incorporated into cardio portions of an exercise class, as during the cardio cool-down. Doing so can be helpful as it allows the participants to become familiar with the size, shape, and feel of the ball before it is used to strength train or stretch. This can also provide a sense of play and inject fun into the class. The use of the ball is really only limited to the imagination and creativity of the instructor designing a class. Ball exercise can be safe, effective, and fun all at once, provided that you understand the principles outlined in this book and obtain specific training on the use of the stability ball from a reputable organization.

Special
Populations

CHAPTER FIVE

S tability ball training can be designed to be appropriate for virtually any population, including all age groups, persons of varying size (height and weight), individuals with orthopedic or post-rehab concerns, and those with chronic medical conditions. As mentioned previously, with such diverse groups the important issue is proper program design for each special population. That requires you to be very aware of the variety of people and conditions you encounter and to understand the unique needs of those groups, as well as movements or positions to avoid to minimize risk of injury. While an in-depth review of this information is beyond the scope of this book, basic guidelines for stability ball use with a variety of special populations are presented below. Note that many of these guidelines are very general and applicable for almost any type of exercise these populations perform.

Pregnant Women

The American College of Obstetricians and Gynecologists (ACOG) has developed guidelines for safe exercise during pregnancy that should be adhered to when teaching ball exercise to pregnant women. Note that exercises from the supine position should be avoided after the fourth month of gestation is completed (American College of Obstetricians and Gynecologists, 1994 & 2002). Stability ball exercises are particularly suited to prenatal women as they focus on strengthening the abdominal, leg, and back muscles, which can help prepare the body for the upcoming rigors of labor. Further, stability ball work during pregnancy assists in maintaining muscle tone and improving strength and endurance to maintain joint stability as the connective tissues relax during pregnancy. The stability ball can be very comfortable for pregnant women, as the shape of the ball readily conforms to body weight, while placing minimal stress on the joints. Squats against a wall with the ball behind the back are an example of using the stability ball to support

the body's natural curvature while performing strengthening exercises. As pregnancy progresses, getting to the floor becomes much more challenging, making the ball an excellent option. The ball also provides added support for seated movements and a rounded surface that comforts and conforms. Remind pregnant exercisers to avoid the Valsalva maneuver (holding breath) during exercises, and advise them to use lighter resistance (30% to 50% of 1 RM) and higher repetitions (12 to 20 per set). The supine incline pelvic tilt can be an effective and challenging abdominal exercise for pregnant women. It enhances muscular control, strength, and postural awareness and may provide the additional benefit of relieving low-back pain. Kegel exercises to strengthen the pelvic floor muscles can also be incorporated during stability ball work. Stretches should be static for pregnant women, and they should avoid deep flexion and joint hyperextension at all times. For more detailed information regarding exercise and pregnancy, refer to *Pre- and Post-Natal Fitness* (Anthony, 2002).

Children

Like all exercise with children, stability ball exercises should emphasize fun and cooperation. Simply sitting on the ball and bouncing and performing push-ups and sit-ups (crunches) on the ball can be fun for kids. Take care to ensure youth are not doing anything harmful or potentially dangerous with the ball, such as bouncing the ball out of control.

Older Adults

Notably, according to the American College of Sports Medicine, the presence of diseases and conditions such as heart disease, stroke, depression, pulmonary disease, renal failure, peripheral vascular disease, osteoporosis, and arthritis are NOT contraindications to exercise (American College of Sports Medicine, 1997, b). Although these conditions, most often seen in older adults, do require modification of the exercise program and monitoring, exercise provides benefits not obtainable with the use of medication alone. For many older adults, the social aspect of exercise, especially prevalent in group fitness, is a significant benefit, aiding in staving off or alleviating feelings of depression, isolation, and loneliness.

With all older adults, whether disease free or not, an extended warm-up and cool-down is advocated. Emphasis on balance training and posture is highly recommended as well. The focus should be on muscle endurance and flexibility training over strength training with significant muscle overload. Speed of movements should be slower with older adults also, and intensity should be added slowly when appropriate. Continually ask older exercisers to monitor their exercise intensities, show them modifications if they are feeling too challenged,

and remind them to discontinue a set early if needed. Become familiar with the most common medications prescribed to older adults and their effects on exercise.

The biggest concern for stability ball use with older adults is balance. Falling is one of the top reasons for hospitalization and death in seniors (due to complications from fracture due to falls). Therefore, ball use must be both careful and controlled (American Council on Exercise, 1998). Because training for balance is one of the best ways these individuals can prepare to avoid falling, balance work is important in terms of functional ability. Bone health is a large concern for the aging population as well. Strength training is effective for maintaining or increasing bone density, as well as muscle mass and strength, all of which aid in the prevention of osteoporosis. Strength work with a balance component, which the stability ball provides, is an ideal way to reduce the risk of falls and possible fractures attributed to those falls (American College of Sports Medicine, 1997; Mazzeo, 1998). Postural instability, which the stability ball helps improve, is another factor involved in frequent falling and fractures. It should be noted that those with osteoporosis in the spine should avoid forward flexion or twisting movements such as squats, crunches, and oblique cross-over moves (Heinrich Rizzo & Knopf, 1999).

Many older adults also experience arthritis to some degree in various joints throughout the body, most commonly the spine, hip, and knee. Stability ball training can build muscle strength and improve muscle function, which can help some seniors cope with arthritis pain. Additionally, the strength gains created with strength training can help improve muscle function and reduce the load on joints, which may help reduce joint pain (Hochberg, 1995). Stretching on the stability ball is helpful for people with arthritis because it can aid in the maintenance of pain-free range of motion in both affected and unaffected joints. People with arthritis need to be very careful of cervical spine alignment during ball work and should avoid exercises that place undue stress on the spine. Neutral wrist alignment is important if additional weights are used with ball exercises for those with arthritis in the wrist. Provide options for ball movements that require supporting the body weight with the hands on the floor for exercisers with arthritis affecting the wrist joints, as excessive wrist flexion should be avoided. Advise exercisers with arthritis in the shoulder to keep the arms at shoulder level and avoid overhead lifting movements. Arthritis in the knee requires that they watch for knee hyperflexion or hyperextension. For this population, closed-chain exercises (feet stay in contact with the ground) are preferred over open-chain exercises (legs move freely in space) to foster functional fitness (American College of Sports Medicine, 1997). Wall squats with the ball behind the back are a more appropriate exercise than seated leg extensions atop the ball. Pay particular attention to placement of the patella over the feet during these closed-chain movements for those with arthritis in the knee. Have clients with arthritis move joints only through their normal, pain-free range of motion during strength or flexibility exercises and avoid exercising when joints are painful, red, or swollen.

Overweight and Obese Individuals

Heavier persons can be appropriately challenged with the stability ball, while at the same time being provided with a soft, comfortable, and supportive prop. Many heavy people have trouble getting down to and up from the floor, and the ball provides an option that minimizes embarrassment. Exercises can be easily modified to provide less challenge if they are too taxing with a simple adjustment in ball placement or widening of the base of support. Ball size should be bigger and less firm to provide more support and comfort in the new or deconditioned overweight exerciser. Provide these individuals with more time to change position, and avoid fast or abrupt moves that require sudden shifting of body weight.

Exercisers with Diabetes

Stability ball work for both the type 1 and type 2 diabetic is appropriate and beneficial. Although there are no specific movements to avoid, the exercise program presented to those with diabetes should minimize stress on the feet, making seated cardiovascular work an excellent alternative to weightbearing activity. Additionally, be aware of the signs and symptoms of hypoglycemia and hyperglycemia. Caution people with diabetes against overworking muscles that will be or have been injected with insulin.

Exercisers with Hypertension or Coronary Heart Disease

Exercisers with either of these conditions should focus on muscle-endurance training, working with less resistance and higher repetitions. Advise them to carefully monitor and maintain exercise intensity at a low to moderate level. While specific stability ball exercises cannot be singled out to avoid, all exercises must be performed with proper breathing techniques. Since stabilizer muscles are in isometric contraction, the tendency is to hold the breath. Remind exercisers with these conditions to use proper breathing techniques and avoid the Valsalva maneuver, because it is extremely high-risk and contraindicated at all times for people with either of these conditions. Both groups should also be careful when lifting the arms over the head or working in a position with the head below the heart. Also, if additional resistance is used for strength work on the ball, it is critical that a relaxed grip be used to hold those

props at all times to avoid elevating blood pressure unnecessarily.

Post-rehab Exercisers

For the purposes of this publication the term post-rehab refers to people who have been released from a physician or therapist's care after rehabilitation from an injury or surgical procedure. Post-rehab training aids in the speed of return to normal functioning following an injury. The stability ball has long been used in this arena because it safely, effectively, and progressively challenges individuals to work with the body as a balanced, coordinated entity. For a person returning from an injury or surgery, develop structural stability and balance around the recovering area and throughout the entire body before returning to pre-injury or pre-surgical levels of activity. The stability ball allows for strength and flexibility work to be performed in very specific movement planes, while balancing and stabilizing the whole body. The post-rehab stage is one of "proceed with caution," with the goal of working toward restoring muscle balance. Advise all post-rehab exercisers to follow the movement restrictions they have obtained from their physician or therapist at all times. Stability ball exercises can easily be designed to accommodate these contraindications to continue the post-rehab exerciser on the road to full recovery.

modifications, 20, 31–33, 67

modified seated hip/glute stretch, 32–33

modified supine incline base position, 20

momentum, avoiding, 31

monitoring, 67

Morris, Mike, 2

Morris, Stephanie, 2

movement speed, 14, 30, 31, 67

multifidus, 10

muscle endurance training, 27, 37–38
    for individuals with hypertension or coronary
    heart disease, 69
    and older adults, 67

muscle strength training, 27, 37–49
    with balance component, for older adults, 67
    modifying, 33
    proper spinal alignment, 39
    upper-body, 45
    warm-up, 26

music, 28

N

neutral neck, 46

neutral pelvis, 17

neutral spine, 13, 15, 16, 68
    and balance, 18
    and posture, 4
    in seated base position, 16–17
    in side-lying position, 22
    for transitions, 24

neutral wrist, 68

new participants, 26

Nottingham, Suzanne, 13

O

oblique cross-over movements, 67

oblique curl
    side-lying, 42
    supine incline, 60

older adults, 67–68

one-leg balance, standing and seated, 58

one-legged squat from the supine incline base
    position using a weighted bar, 47

open-chain exercises, 68

osteoporosis, 67

over-stretching, 51

overweight/obese individuals, 68

P

passive stretches, 49, 52

patella, 68

peak training, 27

pectoralis major, 11

pelvic floor muscles, 10

pelvic tilt, 16, 17, 26
    seated, 59
    supine incline, 20, 59, 66

physical fitness, 13–15

physical therapy, and stability ball, 2

Physioball. *See* stability ball

Pilates, 56

pinched nerve, 16

plank position with and without the ball, 56

plug remover, 6

posterior pelvic tilt, 16, 17

post-rehab exercisers, 69

posture
    and balance, 13, 15–16
    and low-back pain, 12
    and neutral spine alignment, 4
    and older adults, 67
    and stretching, 50, 51

American College of Obstetricians and Gynecologists. (1994). *ACOG Technical Bulletin.* Washington, D.C.: American College of Obstetricians and Gynecologists.

American College of Obstetricians and Gynecologists. (2002). *ACOG Committee Opinion: Exercise During Pregnancy and the Postpartum Period.* Washington, D.C.: American College of Obstetricians and Gynecologists.

American College of Sports Medicine. (1997, a). *ACSM's Facility Standards and Guidelines.* Champaign, Ill.: Human Kinetics.

American College of Sports Medicine. (1997, b). *ACSM's Exercise Management for Persons With Chronic Diseases and Disabilities.* Champaign, Ill.: Human Kinetics.

American College of Sports Medicine. (2000). *ACSM's Guidelines for Exercise Testing and Prescription,* 6/e. Philadelphia, Pa.: Lippincott, Williams & Wilkins.

American Council on Exercise, (1998). *Exercise for Older Adults.* Champaign, Ill.: Human Kinetics.

American Council on Exercise. (2000). *Group Fitness Instructor Manual.* San Diego, Calif.: American Council on Exercise.

American Council on Exercise. (2000). *ACE Fit Fact: Strengthen Your Abdominals with Stability Balls.* San Diego, Calif.: American Council on Exercise.

American Council on Exercise. (2001). Strong abs, strong core, *ACE Certified News,* 7, 4, p 7–9.

Anthony, L. (2002). *Pre- and Post-Natal Fitness.* San Diego, Calif.: American Council on Exercise.

Anders, M. (2001). New study puts the crunch on ineffective ab exercises, *ACE FitnessMatters,* May/June, 9–11.

REFERENCES and Suggested Reading

Bejeck, B. (2000). All about abs. *IDEA Health and Fitness Source*, March, 29–33.

Creager, C.C. & Creswell, B. (2000). Improve core stability using foam rollers. *IDEA Personal Trainer*, July/August, 47–50.

Darragh, A. (1999). Training clients in back and spinal post-rehab. *IDEA Personal Training*, May, 43–51.

Francis, P., Kolkforst, W.W., & Pennucci, M. (2001). EMG evaluation of abdominal exercises. *ACSM's Health & Fitness Journal*, July/August, 10–14.

Ground Control, Inc. (1995). *Resist-A-Ball Manual.* Indianapolis, Ind.: New Times Publishing.

Ground Control, Inc. (1997). *Stretch On The Ball.* Indianapolis, Ind.: New Times Publishing.

Heinrich Rizzo, T. & Knopf, K. (1999). Resistance training for older adults. *IDEA Health and Fitness Source,* June, 32–43.

Hochberg, M.C. (1995). Guidelines for medical management of osteoporosis. *Arthritis and Rheumatism,* 38, 1541–1546.

IDEA. (1999). When you need post-rehab exercise. *IDEA Personal Training,* May, 52.

IDEA. (2001). Fitness programming & equipment trends. *IDEA Fitness Manager,* Oct.

Kahn, J. (2001). Do it right. *Shape Magazine's Fit Pregnancy*, April/May, 44–45.

Mack, C. (1999). Training the post-rehab client. *IDEA Personal Training,* May, 25–41.

Mazzeo, R.S. (1998). ACSM position stand on exercise and physical activity for older adults. *Medicine and Science in Sports and Exercise,* 30, 6, 992–1008.

Morris, M. & Morris, S. (2001,1). Resist-A-Ball Beyond The Basics Workshop, World Fitness IDEA Conference, July.

Morris, M. & Morris, S. (2001,2). Resist-A-Ball Dynamic Flexibility Workshop, World Fitness IDEA Conference, July.

Morris, M. & Morris, S. (2001,3). Resist-A-Ball Gains Weight Workshop, World Fitness IDEA Conference, July.

Nelson, M.E. (1994). Effects of high intensity strength training on multiple risk factors for osteoporotic fractures. *Journal of the American Medical Association,* 272, 1909–1914.

Nottingham, S. (1999). A question of balance. *IDEA Health and Fitness Source,* October, 21–29.

Posner-Mayer, J. (1995). *Swiss Ball Applications for Orthopedic and Sports Medicine.* Longmont, Co.: Ball Dynamics International, Inc.

Sutherland, V. (1999). Yoga gets on the ball. *IDEA Health and Fitness Source,* April, 52–56.

YMCA of the USA. (1995). *YMCA Exercise Instructor Manual.* Champaign, Ill.: Human Kinetics.

YMCA of the USA (2001). *Stability Ball Training: A YMCA Health and Fitness Continuing Education Course.* Chicago, Ill.: YMCA of the USA.

NOTES

NOTES

NOTES

NOTES

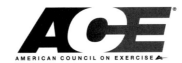

AMERICAN COUNCIL ON EXERCISE

YES, I would like to receive information on the following ACE certifications:

❑ Lifestyle & Weight Management Consultant   ❑ Personal Trainer
❑ Group Fitness Instructor   ❑ Clinical Exercise Specialist

Name _____

Address _____

City_____ State_____ ZIP_____

Home Phone (_____) _____

Work Phone (_____) _____

E-mail _____

AMERICAN COUNCIL ON EXERCISE

YES, I would like to receive information on the following ACE certifications:

❑ Lifestyle & Weight Management Consultant   ❑ Personal Trainer
❑ Group Fitness Instructor   ❑ Clinical Exercise Specialist

Name _____

Address _____

City_____ State_____ ZIP_____

Home Phone (_____) _____

Work Phone (_____) _____

E-mail _____

BUSINESS REPLY MAIL

FIRST-CLASS MAIL   PERMIT NO. 22113   SAN DIEGO, CA

POSTAGE WILL BE PAID BY ADDRESSEE

AMERICAN COUNCIL ON EXERCISE®
PO BOX 910449
SAN DIEGO CA 92191-9961

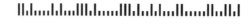

BUSINESS REPLY MAIL

FIRST-CLASS MAIL   PERMIT NO. 22113   SAN DIEGO, CA

POSTAGE WILL BE PAID BY ADDRESSEE

AMERICAN COUNCIL ON EXERCISE®
PO BOX 910449
SAN DIEGO CA 92191-9961

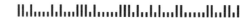